Case Studies and Exercises For
The Resident Assistant

Gregory S. Blimling, Ph.D.
Appalachian State University

KENDALL/HUNT PUBLISHING COMPANY
4050 Westmark Drive   Dubuque, Iowa 52002

Copyright © 1990, 1995 by Kendall/Hunt Publishing Company

ISBN 0–8403–9191–9

Printed in the United States of America
10 9 8 7 6 5 4 3 2 1

Contents

PART I

The History and Foundation of Residence Halls

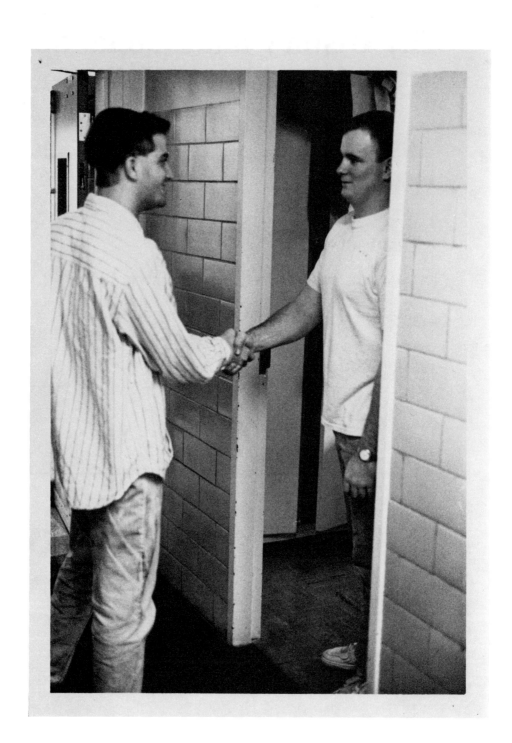

CHAPTER 1

Roles of the RA

1. In the space provided, give four reasons why a person may not want to become an RA.

    1.

    2.

    3.

    4.

2. Give four benefits to an individual that he or she will receive by becoming an RA.

    1.

    2.

    3.

    4.

3. What are the four major roles of an RA?

    1.

    2.

    3.

    4.

4. Which of the above listed roles do you believe is most important, and why?

5. What do you believe is the most unrealistic expectation students have of the RA and why?

6. What do you believe is the most unrealistic expectation college administrators have of RAs and why?

7. What does the author mean in the text when he refers to "conceptual application" skills needed by RAs?

Hall Soccer

Norwood was the RA on four-west. This floor had over half of the residents return to the floor from the previous year. It had the reputation of being rowdy, but also of having a strong sense of community among the residents. The RA on the floor last year was very popular with the residents and made many friends. This was Norwood's first year as an RA, and he wanted to be as well-liked as last year's RA and to do a good job for the university.

About half-way through the second week of the semester, Norwood returned to his floor and found about fifteen of his residents in the hallway and lounge playing hall-soccer. This game had been invented by the residents and involved kicking a soccer ball down the corridor and into the lounge where a goal consisting of the sofa and two chairs had been erected. The game stopped when they saw Norwood. Mike, one of the men who had lived on the floor for the past two years and who was very popular with the other residents, was holding the ball when Norwood appeared. Norwood asked what they were doing, and Mike explained that they were playing hall-soccer. He told Norwood that they played all last year and play the game at least three or four nights a week for several hours at a time. The scuffed walls and broken light fixtures bore proof of Mike's statement.

Questions

1. Norwood does not know what to do. If he stops the game, he believes that he will lose the friendship of most of the residents and may break a floor "tradition" which gives the residents a chance to interact. What would you do if you were Norwood?

2. Is there anything that Norwood could have done to avoid this from happening? If so, what?

What We Value

Claudine was a first-year RA and was active in organizations which opposed abortion. She was a member of a campus group that took an activist stand on opposing abortion. They believed that any effort necessary to save the life of an unborn child was justified. During the summer she had participated in two demonstrations in front of abortion clinics. Her father and mother were also active in the organization, and her mother had been arrested on two occasions for blocking the entrance of an abortion clinic.

Claudine was also very active in a charismatic Christian student organization on campus. She held regular Bible study in her room with some of the other students from the organization and frequently talked about her religious values with the other RAs and other students she knew. She was a warm and personable individual who was well liked in the residence hall. In fact, her warm personality and outgoing style was one of the reasons she was selected as an RA.

When the residence halls opened in the fall semester, Claudine wore a button that said "Abortion is Murder." To every student who obtained a key, she handed an anti-abortion pamphlet that had been produced by the organization to which she belonged. The bulletin board on her floor had a series of photographs showing fetuses that had been aborted at different stages of pregnancy. During the fall semester, her programming effort for her floor was scheduled to consist of a lecture about abortion conducted by two women who headed the local anti-abortion effort and a second program which was billed as a values clarification program directed at promoting abstinence from sex. This latter program was to be conducted by the advisor to the charismatic Christian student organization to which Claudine belonged.

During the first two weeks of class, Claudine went door to door among the residents in the building asking them to sign a petition opposing abortion, asking the university to stop providing information to students about abortions, to stop dispensing birth control pills, and to stop dispensing condoms from the student health center. She and several other students wrote letters to the editor of the student newspaper about abortion. Claudine did not indicate in her letter to the editor that she was an RA. The letter she wrote was signed only with her name and the residence hall where she lived.

In her first floor meeting, Claudine announced to the women on her floor that she was strongly opposed to abortion and saw this as one of the central political themes in her life. She described the abortion issue as a struggle between good and evil and encouraged students who had any questions about this topic to discuss them with her. She said that she knew a lot about this issue and that if anybody was thinking about having an abortion or any of her residents knew anybody who was thinking about abortion to please tell her so she could give them accurate, unbiased, and factual information about abortions. She said that she had been trained as a peer counselor by the university and as an abortion educator by one of the organizations to which she belonged. She was willing and eager to share her time and energy in helping any young women who needed her support and help with handling an unwanted pregnancy.

Questions

1. If you were a student on Claudine's residence hall floor, how would you feel about Claudine asking you to sign a petition?

2. If you or a female friend were considering having an abortion, is Claudine a person you would seek out to discuss this issue? Why or why not?

3. Do you believe that residence life officials should intercede and inform Claudine that she should not be crusading about abortion while she is an RA? Why or why not?

4. Do you believe that Claudine can be objective in counseling students about abortions and in referring them to resources in the counseling center or health center that may have more information on this topic and a different perspective?

5. How would you feel about living on Claudine's floor as one of her residents?

An Unlikely Match

Norwood asked Claudine to go to a party with him off-campus. While at the party, they each saw several people they knew, including several of their residents. The drinking age in the state was 21, and the people who were having the party were over that age and had purchased a keg of beer. Norwood and Claudine were both 19 years old, but both drank alcohol occasionally. The university prohibited alcohol on campus, and RA's were expected to enforce this policy in the residence halls.

Claudine and Norwood both saw several of their under-aged residents drinking alcohol, but neither one commented to the other about it. Claudine stopped and talked with one of her residents. While she was talking, Norwood got himself and Claudine each a beer. Norwood came to where Claudine and her resident were standing and handed her the beer.

Questions

1. What should Claudine do? Should she accept the beer?

2. Do you believe that Claudine should report Norwood to his hall director for drinking alcohol at the off-campus party where some of his residents are also drinking?

3. Do you believe that Claudine should report the illegal use of alcohol by her residents at the off-campus party to her hall director?

4. Would your responses to the above questions be different if Norwood offered Claudine marijuana, and marijuana was being smoked by a number of the party guests including Claudine's residents and Norwood's residents? Why or why not?

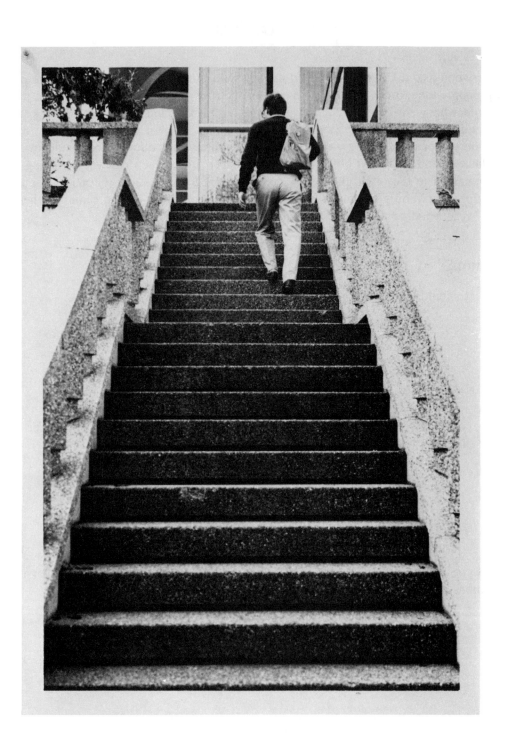

CHAPTER 2

The History of Residence Halls

1. In Europe residence halls flourished until the early 1800's. Give two reasons for the decline of residence halls in continental Europe after the early 1800's.

    1.

    2.

2. What was the single most important reason for the establishment of residence halls in America at the nine original colonial colleges?

3. What is the "residential college concept", and how did it influence the creation of residence halls?

4. Give three reasons for the collapse of the residential college concept in the mid-1800's.

   1.

   2.

   3.

5. What effect did the collapse of the residential college concept have on student housing?

6. Give four reasons for the rebirth of residence halls in the early twentieth century.

   1.

   2.

   3.

   4.

7. What role did women's colleges play in the rebirth of residence halls in the early 1900's?

8. What is the "Student Personnel Point of View"?

9. Give two reasons for the construction of residence halls following World War II.

   1.

   2.

10. What is "ACUHO" and when was it established?

11. Between 1958 and 1968 enrollments at colleges and universities doubled. Give two reasons for this increase.

    1.

    2.

12. What does the term "in loco parentis" mean, and how does it relate to the student-institutional relationship after 1961?

13. Give three reasons for changes in the student-institutional relationship during the 1960's.

    1.

    2.

    3.

14. Give three major differences in the philosophy of working with students in residence halls after the 1960's.

    1.

    2.

    3.

How It Was Then. How It Is Now

Below are lists of some of the policies which governed student behavior in the residence halls of a major state university in 1938. Read the policies for "girls" and "boys" and respond to the questions which follow.

For Girls

A girl's character is always reflected in the way she lives. Your relations among girls in your dormitory will be continually used as a yard stick to the judgment of your true self. To help you achieve a moral standard the Dean of Women, together with the hall house mothers, have offered the following helpful suggestions.

There is a mailbox in every dormitory for the posting of letters. Have all special delivery letters and telegrams addressed to the dormitory and not to boxes.

Read the bulletin boards every day to see if you have a special delivery or telegram, also to observe notices from the Dean of Women regarding special permissions, etc.

Never leave the dormitory overnight without getting special permission from the Dean of Women. A letter from your parents must always be sent to the Dean of Women giving special permission for each time you spend a weekend night in town with friends. Remember to sign a visiting permit card in the dormitory office on return.

Be sure to be in your room for check-up at eight o'clock Monday, Tuesday, Wednesday and Thursday nights. Friday, Saturday and Sunday nights are open night.

Guests are permitted on Friday and Saturday nights. Be sure to register your guest with your housemother. Be sure to introduce your men friends to your housemother. Always rise when an older person speaks to you or enters the room.

Study hour is held Monday, Tuesday, Wednesday, and Thursday nights. Visiting in friends' rooms, radios, and loud talking is not permitted at this time. Turn off lights at 11:15 P.M. unless special permission is received.

Form the habit of signing the hall registers when leaving the campus in the daytime and when leaving the dormitory at night.

Ask your men friends not to call at the dormitory before 1:00 P.M. any day except Sunday.

Do not use the telephone any longer than five minutes. Do not use it during study hour.

Always have your room neat and attractive. Keep the furniture in the room free of all scars and stains. Regard all regulations, keep your rooms neat, and strive to get on the Honor roll. This entitles a girl to an open Wednesday once every three weeks.

Send your laundry out through the chutes of each hall, and call for it at the laundry room in the basement.

Your trunk must be unpacked within 24 hours after your arrival at the University. Put your name on it and send it to the storage room. Trunks are not allowed to remain in the rooms.

Do all your pressing in the pressing rooms. Be careful to always turn off the iron.

Report to the Infirmary in Smith Hall when ill.

Do not keep valuables in the dormitory.

Be sure to have your own room key.

Go to all dormitory meetings.

Go to the candlelight service each Thursday night at 10:00 P.M. in Smith Hall Reception Room.

Budget your time and money carefully.

Wear your hat and gloves to church and afternoon teas. If you are a hostess at an afternoon tea, wear a long afternoon dress, not an evening dress.

Buy your meal tickets from the Auditor's Office in the Alumni Building.

Remember to ask questions when in doubt.

Remember to show good taste in every way on the campus.

*For Boys**

How to live rightly is a problem which all men must face as they enter the University. Each newcomer should try to establish orderly habits immediately. The following information will be of some assistance to men who wish to lead well-balanced lives.

Know your cadet regulations.*

Men who wish to go home frequently over weekends should obtain a letter from their parents authorizing them to do so. Absences from inspections during that time are then automatically excused if intention to take advantage of the weekend privilege is given your first sergeant.

Your first sergeant cannot excuse you from any formation or inspection whatsoever. All excuses accepted by him are first handled through the commandant's office. If you do not want to be refused, never ask him for a privilege he cannot grant.

Study hour is not only a military regulation which must be conscientiously met, but is a time when each man has the opportunity to think of his friends about him who are studying. Be certain that you do not disturb anyone. Absolute quiet begins at 7:30 P.M., and visits are ended.

Your 7:30 A.M. inspections should always be passed by leaving a clean and neat room. Get the habit of hanging up your clothes and get up early enough to sweep thoroughly.

Watch your bulletin board. If your name is always on the right side, you are becoming a success. Strive to make each situation a stepping stone.

When in uniform you are no longer John Doe, but you are a living tribute to the United States of America—any slight in the wearing of your uniform is a blight on your reputation, on your alma mater, and an insult to your country. Be proud, therefore, and wear it correctly.

Questions

1. Give at least five differences between the policies governing women students in the residence halls in 1938 and today.

    1.

    2.

    3.

*Note: The Morell Land Act required that men attending a land grant college complete two years of compulsory enrollment in the Reserve Officer Training Corps (ROTC) as a condition of attendance.

4.

5.

2. Give at least five differences between the policies governing men in the residence halls in 1938 and today.

   1.

   2.

   3.

   4.

   5.

3. Are there any differences in the policies from 1938 governing male students and female students? If so, give examples.

4. After reading the case study, do you denote a differences in the overall philosophy in working with college students evident in the 1938 policies, which is different from the philosophy your institution holds for working with students today? If so, describe the principle differences.

5. Given the brief description of the residence hall policies of 1938, how would you feel about being an RA in 1938? Do you think that the role of the RA has changed and if so, in what ways?

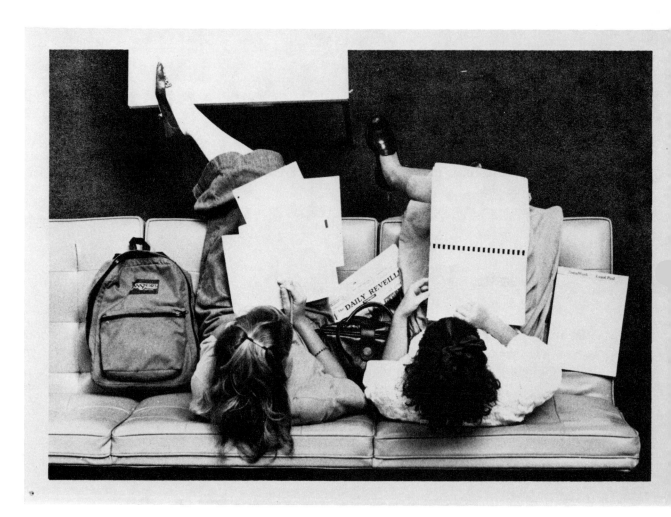

CHAPTER 3

Educational Philosophies
for Residence Halls

1. What is the first responsibility of the director of residence life or housing?

2. Give one characteristic of the "student services approach".

    1.

3. Give one characteristic of the "custodial care and moral development approach".

    1.

4. Give two characteristics of the "student affairs approach".

    1.

    2.

5. Give two characteristics of the "student development approach".

    1.

    2.

6. Give two characteristics of the "Wellness approach."

　　1.

　　2.

7. How would you classify the approach to working with students in residence halls used at your institution?

8. The "Council for the Advancement of Standards for Student Services/Development Program" established a mission for residence life programs. In it are given four goals to accomplish this mission. Briefly, what are three of these goals?

　　1.

　　2.

　　3.

9. Why is it important to the overall educational atmosphere that the residential facilities are well maintained?

10. In the text the author lists what he believes to be educational goals of residence halls. What does he believe is the "primary" goal of residence halls?

How Is He Doing?

Biff was in his second year as an RA at Julian University. He took the job last year because he thought it would look good on his resumé and would help him get into law school. He stayed for the second year because of the resumé and because he liked the extra money it gave him for buying clothes.

Biff was a very conscientious RA. He was meticulous about his record-keeping. Students in his living unit were always checked-in correctly. Biff always filed reports on time and returned all of the surveys and other information the hall director required of him. Regularly he inspected students' rooms for lounge furniture and was prompt about getting light bulbs replaced and items repaired in the living unit. Biff also kept room hours posted on his door. Students who wanted to see him could ''sign up'' for an appointment or could complete a service request form which he kept in a folder on the outside of his room.

Biff was in his room most nights after about 10:00 P.M. or was on duty somewhere in the building. There was no programming requirement in the residence hall, so Biff did not do any. He knew most of the students in his unit and believed that students who needed him would contact him when they needed something. Unless they contacted him, he thought it was best to leave them alone.

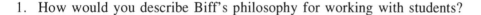

Questions

1. How would you describe Biff's philosophy for working with students?

2. What are Biff's strengths as an RA?

3. What are Biff's weaknesses as an RA?

4. Is Biff's philosophy of working with students in the residence halls consistent with the goals of residence halls as expressed by the "Council for the Advancement of Standards for Student Services/Development Program"? If not, how is it consistent and how is it inconsistent?

How Do You Do Your Job?

1. You have been asked by the residence life department of your institution to talk to a group of new RAs about your philosophy for working with students in the residence halls. Give a brief statement of your philosophy.

2. One of the new RAs asks you to give some examples of group educational and development opportunities you help to provide for students living on your floor. List four.

   1.

   2.

   3.

   4.

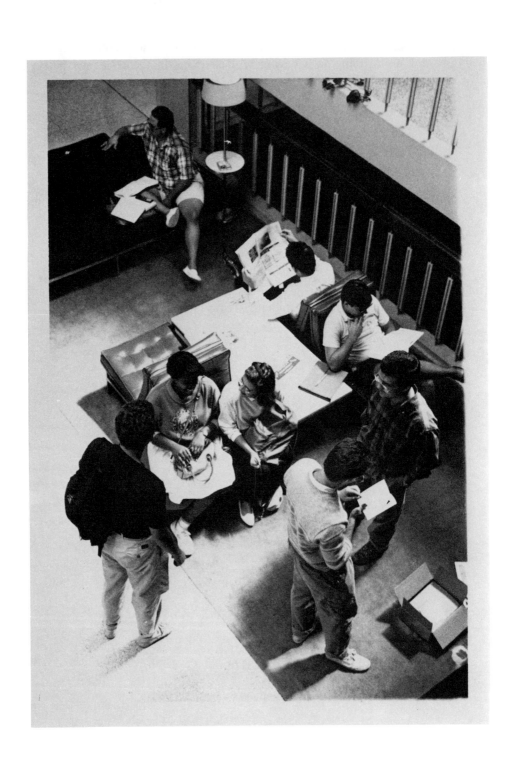

The Influence of Residence Halls on the Development of Students

1. When comparing students who live in residence halls with students who live off-campus (i.e., at home with parents) what advantages do residence hall students obtain over those who live off-campus? List at least six of these differences.

    1.

    2.

    3.

    4.

    5.

    6.

2. Are there any disadvantages to living in the residence halls when comparing residence hall students with students living off-campus? If so, what are they?

3. What influence, if any, does family background have on the differences between students who live in residence halls and students who live at home with parents while attending college?

4. List four methods by which the residence hall experience influences students.

    1.

    2.

    3.

    4.

5. What factor, according to the text, has the greatest influence on a student's (psychosocial) development in college?

6. What influences do a person's college roommate have on his or her development? List three.

    1.

    2.

    3.

7. Give three examples of how the RA influences the development of students in the residence halls.

   1.

   2.

   3.

8. What personal style (counselor or administrator oriented) of the RA is likely to have the greatest influence on students' maturity and satisfaction, and why?

9. List two methods by which students have been assigned to residence halls for the purpose of influencing their intellectual or psycho-social development.

   1.

   2.

10. What is a "living and learning center"?

11. Give five methods for advancing the growth and development of students in the residence halls.

    1.

    2.

    3.

    4.

    5.

12. What is "optimum dissonance"?

13. According to Erikson, what four forms of experience do people need to have in young adulthood to help them develop appropriate adult roles?

    1.

    2.

    3.

    4.

14. When one combines all of the research on residence halls, what are four of the areas in which residence halls seem to have the greatest influence on students?

    1.

    2.

    3.

    4.

15. What influence does the architectural design of a residence hall have on student satisfaction with the residence hall experience and on the social climate of the hall?

The Commuter and the Resident

Missy and Bambi were new freshmen at Tara College. They knew each other from Girls' State where they were roommates for a week. They met again at freshmen orientation. Missy's home was only about fifteen miles from Tara College, so she decided to commute to college and live at home with her parents. She decided to go to Tara College for several reasons, but most of all because it offered her the most financial aid. Her parents both worked. Her mother was a secretary at one of the local high schools, and her father was a roofing contractor. Neither of Missy's parents had the opportunity to attend college. Missy also worked part-time off-campus at a CPA firm answering the telephone and doing general office work. She decided to keep her job while she was attending school for expenses and for personal spending money.

Bambi lived only thirty miles from Tara College, but she decided that she would live on-campus in one of the coed residence halls. Bambi was also receiving some financial aid, but she came to Tara College because both her mother and father were graduates. Like Missy's parents, both of Bambi's parents worked. Her mother worked as a school teacher, and her father was a newspaper reporter with her hometown newspaper. Part of Bambi's financial aid included a work-study job on campus working in the college's admissions office answering the telephone, and doing general office work.

Bambi enjoyed Tara College. She and her roommate became good friends with several other women who lived on their floor. Bambi was elected as the floor representative to residence hall government. She was also active in the hall intramural activities and joined a student organization which supported environmental protection. Bambi had a number of social acquaintances and dated frequently. She also had a season ticket to the campus performing arts program which she and some of the other women from her floor purchased together at the beginning of the year. Academically, Bambi did well. When she had difficulty with an assignment she could usually find someone in her living unit to help her, or she could go to the residence hall library or the main college library.

Missy also enjoyed Tara College, but found it difficult to spend as much time there as she would like. Between classes she would go either to the student union or to the library. Sometimes she would meet someone she knew from class or from high school and they would spend some time talking, but most of the time she either studied on campus or found other things to do between classes. She scheduled her classes to, have as much of the afternoon as free as possible so that she could work at her part-time job off-campus.

Missy joined a campus club in history, but she found it difficult to make their meetings which were on-campus in the evening. She also was not able to make most of their field trips, which were on Saturday, because of her job. Most of her free time was spent with several of her friends from high school who chose not to go to college but to remain at home and work. Missy had a boyfriend whom she dated throughout most of high school and who was working as an apprentice electrician with a local construction contractor. She dated him exclusively. Academically, Missy was doing well, but she spends at least four to five hours each night to keep up in her classes. The branch library is about five miles from her home. It contains some of the materials she needs as references. She can use this library for references or she can drive to campus to use the main college library. Professors are usually available by appointment or after class to help her with assignments, and she tries hard to anticipate any problems with the assignments far enough in advance so that she can make arrangements to see one of her professors about the problem.

Questions

1. Who do you believe has the best chance of graduating from college, Missy or Bambi? Why?

2. In what important ways are Missy's college experience different from those of Bambi?

3. What could Missy do to improve the quality of her college experience?

Friends

Buddy and Floyd were assigned together as roommates at Big South University. They met for the first time during the fall semester when they moved into the residence hall. Floyd was a National Merit Scholarship recipient and was given a full tuition waiver at Big South University. The scholarship would be continued as long as Floyd maintained a 3.0 (scale of 4.0 = A) grade point average.

Buddy was a reasonably good student in high school but he was not nearly the caliber of student that Floyd was. Buddy was an outstanding athlete in school, and was voted the most popular guy in his senior class. Everyone liked Buddy, and Buddy liked everyone. He was a nice looking young man and had a very active social life. One of Buddy's skills was organizing and having parties. His good interpersonal and social skills made him the quintessential host or party guest.

Floyd admired Buddy. Although Floyd was reasonably good looking, he lacked the social confidence and poise which seemed to come so naturally to Buddy. Because of Buddy's interpersonal skills, Floyd and Buddy's room became the social focus of activities on the floor. There was always someone in their room talking, watching a football game, or playing cards. Seldom did any of this activity break up before 1:00 A.M. During times the room was occupied by others, Buddy was either talking on the telephone, or Floyd was taking messages for him. Buddy was also thinking about pledging a fraternity, and two fraternities were rushing him very hard. They also rushed Floyd, but he thought it might be because he was Buddy's roommate. This simply added to the confusion. At least one night each weekend, Floyd found himself sleeping in either the floor lounge or in someone else's room, because Buddy usually brought his date back to the room where they would spend most of the night together.

Although Floyd realized that all of this activity was detracting from his school work, he liked Buddy and the other men on the floor. He wanted to be a part of the group and enjoyed the attention he got from the people who were constantly in and out of his room. This experience did have some positive benefits for Floyd. He felt more self-confident, was more comfortable in groups, and had made some friends. Floyd's social life had also improved. He had been on several double dates with Buddy and his girlfriend, and was beginning to develop a relationship with one woman in particular.

Mid-term grades were sent home to Floyd's and Buddy's parents. Floyd's grade point average at mid-term was 2.2. Buddy's g.p.a. was also 2.2, which he thought was fine. His parents, knowing Buddy's strengths and weaknesses, thought it was acceptable. Floyd's parents, though, were very concerned. They realized that Floyd would lose his scholarship if his grades did not improve. They called the Dean of Students at Big South University, who called the hall director, who talked to Buddy and Floyd's RA. The hall director wanted the RA's recommendation on what to do, if anything, about Floyd, his new life-style, and his roommate.

Questions

1. If you were Floyd and Buddy's RA what recommendation(s) would you make to the hall director about Floyd?

2. Is Buddy at fault for the negative study environment in Buddy and Floyd's room? Why or why not?

3. What positive benefits have there been for Floyd, and do these outweigh the poor academic performance?

4. Floyd's parents have suggested that he be moved to a "study floor" in another building where study hours are strictly enforced, or that he be given a single room some place on campus. What do you think about these ideas?

PART II

Understanding and Working with College Students

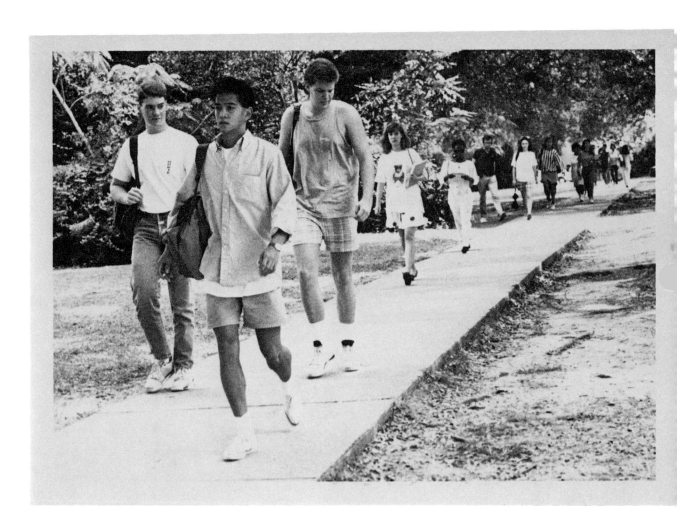

CHAPTER 5

The Growth and Development
of College Students

1. In section A, Chickering's seven vectors of development in college are given. Section B contains a list of developmental issues students exhibit during the college years. Match the vectors with the behaviors by placing the appropriate vector letters (A–G) in the space provided to the left of the developmental issue. Vectors are used more than once.

Section A: Chickering's Seven Vectors
    A. Developing Competence
    B. Managing Emotions
    C. Developing Autonomy
    D. Establishing Identity
    E. Freeing Interpersonal Feelings
    F. Developing Purpose
    G. Developing Integrity

Section B: Developmental Issues
    _____ 1. A freshman who refuses to talk with parents
    _____ 2. A junior who is spending all of his free time with his girlfriend
    _____ 3. A freshman who is concerned with fitting in with the other students
    _____ 4. A sophomore who cannot control his temper
    _____ 5. A sophomore male who is homophobic
    _____ 6. A junior who is searching for a college major
    _____ 7. A student from the student judicial committee who gets caught shoplifting in the campus bookstore
    _____ 8. A freshman who is worried about being as intelligent as the other students in his/her classes.
    _____ 9. A sophomore student who wants to live in an off-campus apartment
    _____ 10. A freshman who continually violates college regulations
    _____ 11. A sophomore who enters a college sponsored co-op program in which he or she alternately works one semester and attends college one semester
    _____ 12. A student who announces her engagement
    _____ 13. A freshman who is overly concerned about her appearance
    _____ 14. A student who spends much of his time proving to others how much he can drink, how tough he is, and how brave he can be
    _____ 15. A freshman who is concerned because he cannot decide on a college major

2. Define the term "growth" as it is used in the text.

3. Define the term "development" as it is used in the text.

4. Explain what is meant by the term "developmental crisis."

5. Erikson states that development is driven by two forces. What are these two forces?

    1.

    2.

6. Give three characteristics associated with psychosocial development.

   1.

   2.

   3.

7. Give three characteristics associated with cognitive development.

   1.

   2.

   3.

8. Cognitive development occurs through a process of adaptation. What are the two adaptive processes in cognitive development and how is each defined?

   1.

   2.

9. Perry identified three major periods of cognitive development in college students. Identify these three periods.

   1.

   2.

   3.

10. Kohlberg identified six stages of moral development. What are these six stages?

   1.

   2.

   3.

   4.

5.

6.

11. In Kohlberg's theory of moral development most college students are found in what stage of moral development?

12. What are the three major stages of moral development in women identified in Gilligan's theory?

Lucy

Lucy was a freshman at State University. She was a little overwhelmed by the size of the University which had 40,000 students and about 7,000 faculty and other employees. Her hometown had only 7,000 people in it, and her entire high school graduating class had fewer students in it than the number of women living on her residence hall floor. Lucy came to State because it was the land grant institution and offered the state's only agriculture degree.

Lucy did not make friends easily. She was somewhat shy and hoped that the experience of going to college would help her with her shyness. Lucy's scheduled roommate never showed, leaving Lucy with a single room and the possibility of having someone assigned to the room later in the semester. Lucy kept to herself the first two weeks of school. She lived in a residence hall at the end of a long double-loaded corridor which had about forty-five women on it.

By the end of the first month of classes, Lucy had still not made any friends in the residence hall. She got up in the morning, went to classes, and came back to her room and stayed there. She was very unhappy and was thinking about going home. The residence hall handbook instructed students who were having a problem in school to first consult their RA. She went to the RA's room to tell her RA that she thought she wanted to leave school and wanted to know what procedure she needed to follow to withdraw from State University.

Questions

1. If you were Lucy's RA, how would you counsel her?

2. Is there anything that Lucy's RA could have done to have helped Lucy make friends early in the semester? If so, what?

3. What are the major developmental issues Lucy seems to be confronting?

4. How can the RA help Lucy address these developmental issues?

Right Meets Left

Hans is a freshman who lives in a single room on the second floor in an all male residence hall of about 300 men. His RA is Clyde. Hans went to a military high school and is very precise about everything. He keeps his closet and his other belongings in impeccable order. Hans has very conservative political views and is active in the College Republicans and the Young Americans for Freedom. Proudly displayed in his room is an American flag and a photograph of a U.S. Marine Corps recruiting poster. Although he has not yet decided if he wants to join ROTC, he is giving it serious thought. On most topics Hans has a strong opinion. The classes he likes best are math and science. He likes philosophy and history least because the professors in these courses won't give him a ''straight answer'' to his questions. Hans does not fit in with most of the other students on the floor and has become somewhat of a joke.

Asher is a freshman who lives on the same residence hall floor as Hans—about five rooms from Hans's. Asher is quite different from Hans. He wears blue jeans with holes in the knees, one silver earring, and usually a T-shirt with the name of some type of ''heavy-metal'' rock group on it. Asher believes that everyone should have the right to do his or her own thing. He does not like most of the rules in the residence hall but abides by them because he does not want to get into trouble. Asher has an American flag which he uses as a rug in his room. Asher intends to major in philosophy. He likes philosophy because he believes that it allows everyone to have their own opinions about things.

One day Hans was in his room studying when he heard rather loud heavy-metal music coming from Asher's room. When he went to Asher's room, the door was open and he saw Asher dancing on the American flag which was being used as a rug. Screaming above the music, Hans got Asher's attention. He asked Asher to turn down the music, which Asher did. Hans then told Asher that he thought Asher was a degenerate for dancing on the American flag and that only a communist drug fiend would ever show such disrespect for the flag. Asher acknowledged that he did occasionally use drugs and had not yet decided if he was a communist or an anarchist. He told Hans that when he decided what he was, he would get back to him but until then, Hans could ''stay the hell out of his way.'' Some words and threats were exchanged, and Hans left and went back to his room, whereupon Asher turned his music up twice as loud.

That night someone forced pennies against the lock to Hans's room, making it impossible for him to open it from the inside. Bottle rockets and shaving cream were then shot under the door, followed by a bucket of water under the door. When Clyde, the RA, returned to his floor he found Hans screaming in his room and pounding on the door. There was no one in the hall, but most of the residents were awake and in their rooms with their doors open. Most were laughing. When Clyde let Hans out of his room, Hans was so angry, he did not know what to do with himself. He started down to Asher's room to confront Asher, who he suspected of the vandalism. Asher did not answer the door, but stayed inside listening to his music.

Questions

1. If you were the RA what would you do?

2. Based on the facts of the case study, what would be your best guess as to Hans's stage of cognitive development using Perry's scheme and why?

3. Based on the factors of the case study, what would be your best guess as to Asher's stage of cognitive development using Perry's scheme and why?

4. Is there anything that could be done by the RA to facilitate the cognitive growth of both students?

5. How do you think the RA can best resolve the conflict between Asher and Hans before it escalates into more serious pranks?

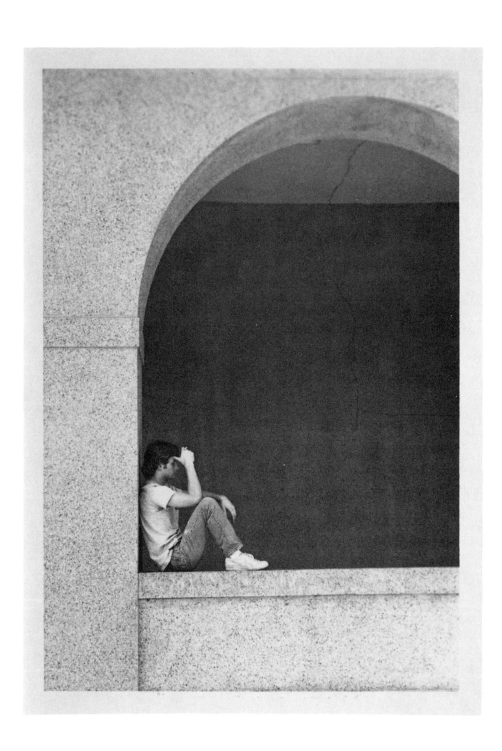

CHAPTER 6

Adjustment Problems in the College Years

1. In the space provided, indicate if the adjustment problem is most likely to occur in the freshman year (F), the sophomore or junior year (S/J), or the senior year (S).

_____ 1. homesickness
_____ 2. problems with parents
_____ 3. intimacy
_____ 4. marital plans
_____ 5. doubt over whether or not to continue in college
_____ 6. authoritarian personality
_____ 7. boyfriend/girlfriend conflicts
_____ 8. pressure to live off-campus
_____ 9. stabilization of a vocational preference
_____ 10. sex-role identification problem

2. When a freshman begins living in a residence hall, he or she goes through an adaptation phase. How long is this period and what is its importance to the RA?

3. What roles do the architectural or environmental design of a residence hall play in the maintenance of peer groups?

4. Historically, why have freshmen women had a more difficult time establishing autonomy than have men?

5. In the freshmen year, most students experience a "break in the child-parent relationship." What is meant by this phrase and what is its function in a student's development?

6. What are some of the advantages and disadvantages to assigning freshmen to live in the same residence halls with upper-class students (i.e., sophomores, juniors and seniors)?

7. Why do most men often have more difficulty with issues of emotional development than do women?

8. Identify three academic skills and three personal skills freshmen learn in their first year of college.

Academic Skills

   1.

   2.

   3.

Personal Skills

   1.

   2.

   3.

9. If new roommates react negatively to each other when they first meet, what are some of the things the RA can do in subsequent weeks to help the two students adjust?

10. If roommates continue to have problems after two or three weeks, what is likely to be the best course of action and why?

11. What is "sophomore slump" and what are some of the reasons it may occur?

12. What is the primary reason students want to move from the residence hall into an apartment during the sophomore or junior year? Do you think there is a good educational reason for letting students move from the residence halls after the first or second year? Explain why or why not.

Crimes of the Heart

David was a criminal justice major. He enjoyed the first year of college, but the second year was just not as interesting. It seemed like it would take forever for him to finish the core course requirements of his college. He had taken only two courses in his major, and he enjoyed them. The foreign language requirement and the advanced math requirement were giving him the most difficulty. He had dropped both last semester because he could not keep up with the class.

If it were not for Carol, he might have just dropped out of college and joined a police force someplace. Carol was a student he met at the beginning of the fall semester, and they had been dating regularly since the second week of the fall semester.

One night David returned to the residence hall and saw Carol standing in front of the hall talking with another man. They were laughing and seemed to be having a good time. David was jealous. He watched them for awhile, and then approached them. He was polite, but it was evident that he found this situation stressful. When the other young man left, David began to quiz Carol about him. His questions were so intense that Carol got angry and told David that she wasn't some criminal and to stop the "third degree" questioning. David got angry and the two had a major fight which ended in Carol telling David she never wanted to see him again.

David returned to his room, frustrated and upset. His roommate tried to console him with statements like "you were too good for her," and "there are alot of fish in the sea—learn to play the field."

During the following week, David tried to call Carol at least a dozen times. She spoke to him only once. She told him that it was not just the fight they had that made her break-off the relationship, but there were some other things that also bothered her. She told him that he was "a nice guy" and that she hoped that they could just be "good friends." David fell into a deep depression. He stopped eating and stopped going to classes.

David came back to the room one afternoon and told his roommate that he had decided to drop-out of college and was giving serious thought to joining the Marine Corps. He planned to meet with a recruiter tomorrow. He was not going to tell his parents, because it was his decision and he didn't want them to try and interfere.

David's roommate was concerned and went to talk with the RA. He told the RA the whole story.

Questions

1. If you were David's RA what would you do?

2. What developmental issues is David confronting?

3. Do you think that David should be allowed by the college to withdraw and join the Marine Corps without someone from the college talking with David's parents?

4. What adjustment problems is David experiencing?

5. List three things the RA could do to help David with his personal adjustment.

   1.

   2.

   3.

6. What are some of the potentially positive and negative outcomes of David's decision to leave college and join the Marine Corps?

Student Problems: Old and New

Rhoda Orme was acting as a "dormitory counselor" (Hall Director) at Barnard College after a number of years working as an instructor and academic dean at Bradford Junior College. In 1950 she wrote *Counseling in Residence Halls*. From her experience she observed that the most common student problems among freshmen women in 1950 were the following:

1. Having to supervise personally one's own activities without being checked on, as at home

2. Feeling lonely because one is afraid at first to talk confidentially to new friends

3. Finding oneself to be a little frog in a big pond, the opposite of the situation in a small-town high school

4. Finding out that college life is not as glamorous as one imagined

5. Trying to decide what to do about an unlikable girl who sticks close

6. Wasting too much time in "bull sessions" and bridge games, and then letting work pile up because there is no check-up in class

7. Resisting the temptation to ask advice about many details from a roommate, as one did from family at home

8. Not being able to figure out "what the professor wants"

9. Finding it hard to compete with girls who have had wide social experiences

Questions

1. Are these problems of the 1950's still problems for most students today? If so, which three do you believe are the most significant problems? If you do not believe these issues are problems for most students, what do you believe has changed so that these issues are no longer major concerns?

2. Make a list of the five problems you believe are most common among freshmen.

    1.

    2.

    3.

    4.

    5.

3. Do you believe that male and female freshmen have different kinds of problems in the freshman year? If so, what are these differences?

4. Choose any **three** of the common student problems Rhoda Orme observed and identify the psycho-social or cognitive developmental issue it reflects.

   1.

   2.

   3.

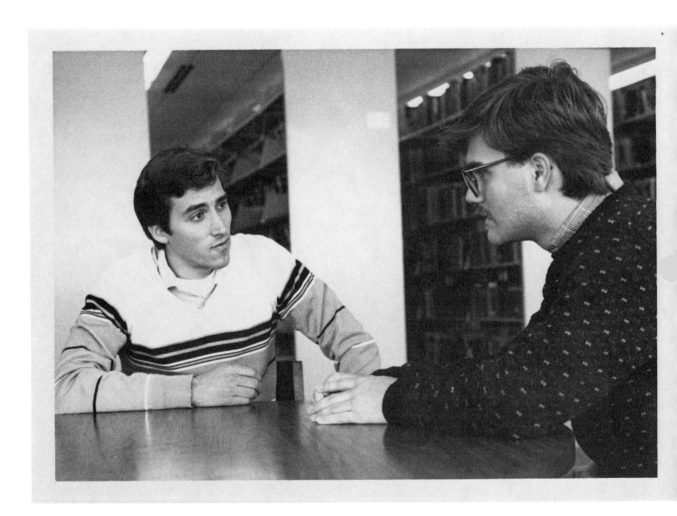

CHAPTER 7

Peer Counseling

1. Below is a list of situations you might encounter as an RA. From the information provided, indicate in the space to the left if you would: (A) initiate a counseling contact with the student, (B) contact and counsel with the student and refer the student to the hall director, (C) contact and counsel with the student and refer the student to the campus mental health or counseling center, (D) not take any action at this time.

_____ 1. Paul is very depressed about breaking up with a girl he has been dating for the past year. He seems depressed and angry about the situation.

_____ 2. Violet is spending much of her time at college bars. Her usual pattern of behavior is to get intoxicated and then bring a man back to her single room in the residence hall and spend the night with him. She has been bringing a different man back to her room almost every night.

_____ 3. Bud has the reputation of being very difficult. He is suspicious of others and given to violent, unexplained outbursts of emotion.

_____ 4. Lucy did not do as well as she expected on her mid-term grades. She was expecting to get a 3.5 grade point average or better, and she received a 3.0. She thinks her parents will be angry with her and has been depressed most of the day.

_____ 5. Carruth lost his brother in an automobile accident earlier in the semester. He seemed fine when he first returned to the residence hall, but recently he has retreated from activities with other students and has been keeping to himself.

_____ 6. You suspect that one of your residents, Ernest, is gay because you saw him walking out of a gay bar near the campus and passionately embrace and kiss another male. You are almost certain that his roommate is not gay and that he does not know that Ernest is.

_____ 7. Barbara has been spreading rumors about another student on the floor. This gossip is malicious, and if it gets back to the person who she is talking about, it would both hurt her feelings and result in some form of retaliation.

_____ 8. Frances and three other women from your living unit went through sorority rush together. Frances was the only one not to get a bid to a sorority.

_____ 9. You are in the shower room when you observe one of your residents who is pledging a fraternity remove his clothes and reveal a series of welts across his buttocks and thighs.

_____ 10. Nancy took a long weekend and went on a three-day retreat with a religious group of some kind. She returned to the residence hall and has been telling everyone that she has experienced a revelation in her life. She has given away all of her records and CDs and has been spending most of her time with people from this religious group or reading the Bible.

_____ 11. Norman has been very depressed for the past two weeks after breaking up with his girlfriend. He has stopped going to classes and has recently given away his most prized possessions. The past couple of days he has appeared much happier.

_____ 12. Sheila is white and her new roommate is black. It is the first week of school, and the two never seem to do anything together. They eat with different groups in the cafeteria and do not appear to be spending much time together.

2. Define an "open-ended" question and give an example of one.

3. What is the first step in the counseling exchange with a student and what kinds of physical steps can you take to set the environment for this exchange?

4. What is the proper counseling posture and why?

5. What are the five stages of counseling as defined in the text?

    1.

    2.

    3.

    4.

    5.

6. What is the goal of the helping skills encounter with students?

7. Give three examples of counseling techniques you use in the listening stage of counseling.

    1.

    2.

    3.

8. What are the four steps to be accomplished in the problem identification and analysis stage?

    1.

    2.

    3.

    4.

9. When should you make a referral of a student to professional counseling?

10. What are three of the behavioral signs which may indicate a need for professional counseling?

    1.

    2.

    3.

11. How does "advising" differ from "counseling"?

12. Give three reasons why it is necessary for the RA to establish the behavioral expectations for the living unit early in the academic year.

    1.

    2.

    3.

Understanding Yourself

INSTRUCTIONS: Under each category circle all of the statements with which you **disagree.**

A. RACE

  1. I would have a person of another race as a friend
  2. I would have a person of another race as a roommate
  3. I would date a person of another race
  4. I would consider marrying a person of another race
  5. As an RA I can be objective in working with a student of another race

B. RELIGION

  1. I would have a person of another religion as a friend
  2. I would have a person of another religion as a roommate
  3. I would date a person of another religion
  4. I would consider marrying a person of another religion
  5. As an RA I can be objective in working with students who have different religious beliefs than my own

C. ABORTION

  1. I would have a person who had an abortion as a friend
  2. I would have a person who had an abortion or who encouraged his girlfriend to have an abortion as a roommate
  3. I would date a person who had an abortion or who encouraged his girlfriend to have an abortion
  4. I would consider marrying a person who had an abortion or who encouraged his girlfriend to have an abortion
  5. As an RA I can be objective in working with students who have had an abortion or who encouraged their girlfriends to have an abortion

D. OVERWEIGHT

  1. I would have an obese person as a friend
  2. I would have an obese person as a roommate
  3. I would date an obese person
  4. I would consider marrying an obese person
  5. As an RA I can be objective in working with obese students

E. HOMOSEXUALITY

  1. I would have a homosexual person as a friend
  2. I would have a homosexual person as a roommate
  3. I would date a person of the same gender
  4. I would consider engaging in a long-term sexual relationship with a person of the same gender
  5. As an RA I can be objective in working with homosexual students

F. DRUGS (Illegal Drugs, i.e., marijuana, cocaine, speed)

   1. I would have a person who used drugs as a friend
   2. I would have a person who used drugs as a roommate
   3. I would date a person who used drugs
   4. I would consider marrying a person who used drugs
   5. As an RA I can be objective in working with students who used drugs outside of the residence halls

G. ANTI-AMERICANISM (Defined as a strong dislike of the United States government, capitalism, and critical of American culture)

   1. I would have an anti-American international student as a friend
   2. I would have an anti-American international student as a roommate
   3. I would date an anti-American international student
   4. I would consider marrying an anti-American international student
   5. As an RA I can be objective in working with anti-American international students

H. PHYSICALLY HANDICAPPED (i.e., paraplegic)

   1. I would have a physically handicapped student as a friend
   2. I would have a physically handicapped student as a roommate
   3. I would date a physically handicapped student
   4. I would consider marrying a physically handicapped student
   5. As an RA I can be objective in working with a physically handicapped student

I. BLINDNESS

   1. I would have a blind student as a friend
   2. I would have a blind student as a roommate
   3. I would date a blind student
   4. I would consider marrying a blind student
   5. As an RA I can be objective in working with a blind student

Fourth Down and Long

Juan is a new RA in a men's residence hall. He is responsible for a floor of approximately forty men. He wants to do a good job as an RA and wants to be liked by his residents. The first week of school he organized a large group of his residents to go off-campus with him to a private club where they serve beer or wine to people over eighteen—which is legal in private clubs in his state. He also had men from his floor in his room most of the time playing cards and socializing.

At the beginning of the year, Juan told his residents that he wanted them to have a good time in college and that he would always be available to them. He told them that university regulations did not permit alcohol in undergraduate residence halls, that marijuana and all other drugs were forbidden, and that there should be quiet hours each school evening from 8:00 P.M. to 8:00 A.M. He told his residents that he was not going to be a "cop", and as long as he did not see anything, they would be all right.

Juan would usually watch Monday night football in the room of his former roommate who lived on another floor in the same building. In the privacy of his roommate's room, he and his old roommate would usually have a few beers while they enjoyed the game. About half-way into the semester, his roommate got ill and was not able to watch Monday night football with Juan. Juan went to the library Monday night to study for mid-term exams. He returned about 10:00 P.M. When he entered the building, he met the duty RA who said he got a complaint about the noise on Juan's floor and was on his way to check on it.

When the two RAs entered the floor, they saw about twenty of Juan's residents in the floor lounge drunk and yelling about the football game they were watching on TV. One of the older residents purchased a pony-keg of beer with money he collected from residents. When the duty RA asked what was going on, he was told to stop interrupting the game, that they do this every Monday night and for him to mind his own business.

Questions

1. Should the duty RA report this unauthorized party and violation of the alcohol regulations to the hall director? Why or why not?

2. Juan asks the duty RA not to report the situation to the hall director because the hall director has had other complaints about him and Juan is afraid that the hall director will fire him. Juan promises he will talk to his residents about the situation. If you were the duty RA, would you still report the situation? Why or why not?

3. What should Juan do? Should he report the students to the hall director? Why or why not?

4. If Juan reports the students, he is afraid the residents will stop liking him and will not come to him when they have problems. Do you think Juan is correct? Why or why not?

5. Do you think it is possible to be both liked and respected by students when you are an RA? If you answer yes, explain how to do this. If you answer no, explain why this is not possible.

6. What could Juan have done to avoid this situation?

The Social Outsider

Ruby is a sophomore in a large state university. She selected the university because it had a program in fashion design in which she was interested. Ruby does not have good social skills and frequently seems to say the wrong thing at the wrong time. The other women on her residence hall floor don't like her. She just doesn't fit in. The clothes she wears are "exotic." She overuses make-up, and her personal hygiene needs attention. Her roommate transferred to another room as soon as she had the opportunity. She couldn't stand being around Ruby because of Ruby's lack of personal hygiene and the immense clutter that Ruby had in the room.

Ruby's attitude about the other women on the floor is that, "If they don't like me, I won't like them." She ignores them. She goes to class alone, eats alone, and comes back to her room, closes the door, and watches TV alone. Needless to say, Ruby does not date and does not fit in well with the other students who are in the fashion design program.

Ruby became increasingly depressed. She made a decision that she needed to make some changes in her life but didn't possess the information and personal skills necessary to address these issues. As she became increasingly depressed, she started binge eating. The more depressed she became, the more junk food she consumed. She knew that she did not want to get any fatter than she was and that this might interfere with her career goals in fashion design.

One night after dinner, the RA entered the bathroom and heard Ruby vomiting in one of the bathroom toilet stalls. When the RA asked Ruby if she was sick, Ruby indicated that she was ill. Two nights later, the RA saw Ruby enter the bathroom after dinner and, after waiting a few minutes, followed her in. Again she heard Ruby vomiting in a toilet stall. She asked Ruby if she was ill, and again Ruby indicated that she was.

Questions

1. What should Ruby's RA do, if anything?

2. How would you go about making a counseling contact with Ruby? What are some of the open-ended questions you could use to help Ruby discuss some of the issues she is probably facing?

3. List three things that you could say to Ruby or do for Ruby that would help her seek professional counseling to address what appears to be bulimic behavior.
    1.

    2.

    3.

4. The other women on the floor often make fun of Ruby. Should the RA say anything to the other women on the floor about their behavior toward Ruby? What should the RA say or do, if anything?

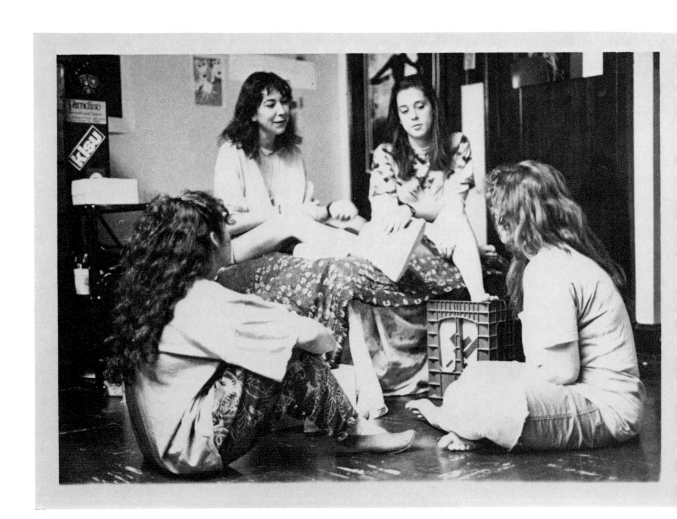

CHAPTER 8

Interpersonal Communication

1. Identify the three levels of communication and give an example of each.

    1.

    2.

    3.

2. Why does the residence hall environment lend itself to the establishment of interpersonal relation-ships?

3. Give two examples of situations that stimulate interpersonal communication.

    1.

    2.

4. When are interpersonal relationships most likely to occur?

5. What are the two steps to empathizing?

    1.

    2.

6. Why is it often difficult for the RA to establish interpersonal relationships with students in his or her living unit?

7. List two advantages and two disadvantages to RAs developing close personal relationships with students in their living units.

    Advantages

    1.

    2.

    Disadvantages

    1.

    2.

8. Give two advantages and two disadvantages to RAs developing close personal relationships with other RAs.

Advantages

1.

2.

Disadvantages

1.

2.

Strangers

Titus was in his third year of being an RA and planned to graduate at the end of spring semester. He was somewhat reluctant to return to being an RA the third year, but he needed the money and was close friends with four of the RAs from last year who were also returning.

Titus was assigned as an RA to the same floor he had last year. Most of his residents did not return. About eighty percent of the residents were new. Of the men who did return, Titus knew only four well. Titus went through the motions of introducing himself to the new residents, but his heart was just not in the RA position. He was more interested in finishing college and getting a job. Titus spent most of his free time with the RAs he knew from last year. Although he stayed in his room during duty-nights, usually one of his RA friends would be in his room with him, or his door would be closed and he would be studying.

About mid-way through the semester, several of Titus' residents complained to the hall director that they were not getting notices of what was taking place in the residence hall and that their RA was never there. They said that the only time they ever saw him was at dinner, and he always sat at the "RA table."

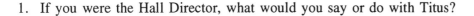

Questions

1. If you were the Hall Director, what would you say or do with Titus?

2. Should the Hall Director fire Titus for not doing his job? Why or why not?

3. The hall director tells Titus that he has the rest of the fall semester to make friends with most of the men on his floor. He said that he will be evaluating his performance, and wants Titus to submit a plan on how he intends to do this. Develop a plan for Titus to follow that will help him establish friendships and trust with most of the men in his living unit.

Brenda

Brenda was a new resident on Carmen's floor. Brenda lived at home the first semester of her freshman year and decided to live in the residence hall at the insistence of her parents, who were hoping that this experience would help her meet more people. As the RA on the floor, Carmen knew that most of the friendships among the women were formed in the first semester. Brenda was the only new person on the floor, and worse yet, she was assigned to live with Claudia. Although Claudia was assigned to live in the room, she was living with her boyfriend off-campus. Claudia did not want her parents to know and kept the room so that her parents wouldn't find out where she was really living. She would usually return to the room once a day to check her messages on her answering machine and check her mail.

Brenda was shy and somewhat introverted. She did not make friends easily. The experience of living in a residence hall intimidated her a little, however, she was willing to give it a try. The hall director spoke with Brenda's parents when she moved in. They confided their concerns about their daughter to the hall director. The hall director assured them that she and her RAs would do everything they could to help Brenda get adjusted and make new friends. The day Brenda moved in, the hall director came to Carmen's room and asked her to help Brenda adjust to the residence hall. She confided in Carmen the parents' concerns and asked Carmen to do everything she could to help Brenda.

Questions

1. What are some of the concerns Brenda might have about moving into the residence hall?

2. If you were Carmen, what would you do to help Brenda adjust to the residence hall?

3. What things could Carmen do to help Brenda make friends when friendship groups were already established on the floor and everyone seemed occupied with their own schedules?

4. Do you think the RA should talk to Claudia about her deceiving her parents? Why or why not? Should the RA tell the hall director? Why or why not?

Confrontation and Crisis Management

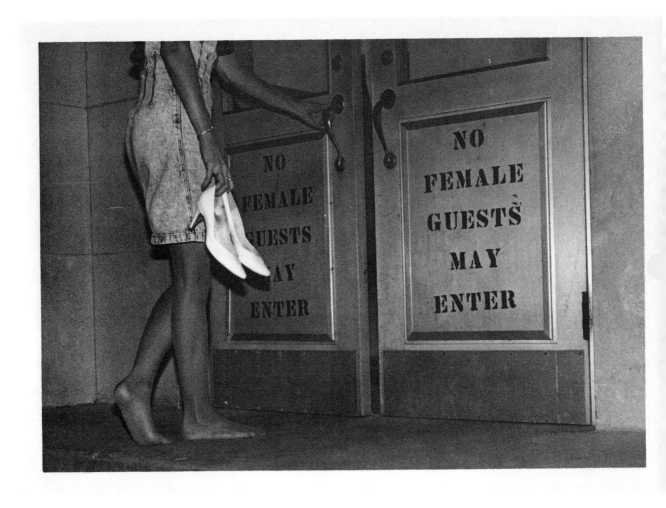

CHAPTER 9

Behavior Problems, Confrontations, and Counseling

1. There are five types of regulations universities enforce. Identify these five types.

    1.

    2.

    3.

    4.

    5.

2. How is assertive communication different from aggressive communication?

3. Give three typical responses a student might give when approached about a behavioral violation.

    1.

    2.

    3.

4. The text says that the RA should achieve a meaningful dialogue with the student. What is meant by a "meaningful dialogue" and what are some of the do's and don't's for achieving it?

5. There are only three reasons given in the text for confronting an intoxicated person. What are they?

   1.

   2.

   3.

6. In the case of confronting an intoxicated person with a disciplinary problem, what is the immediate goal?

7. Why is it not a good idea to accept information from students under the condition you not tell anyone else?

8. What are some of the problems associated with openly expressing to your residents your objections to policies?

9. Why are the first few weeks of the fall semester important in avoiding disciplinary problems in your living unit?

10. Define the terms "rationalization" and "projection".

    Rationalization:

    Projection:

11. Why is the follow-up step important in the disciplinary encounter?

12. Give three ways the hall director can assist you in working with disciplinary problems in your living unit.

   1.

   2.

   3.

The Viking

Howell is a second semester freshman living on the fourteenth floor of North Tower. His RA is Franco. Howell came to State University to play football, but was not quite good enough to make the team. His nickname on the 14th floor is "The Viking." He got this nickname as the result of his large size, table manners, temper, and ability to consume very large quantities of beer. Howell is not much of a student. This semester he is only enrolled for six hours of course work, after having dropped nine hours because he was not doing well academically.

Franco was on duty Friday night and went to sleep about 1:00 A.M., hoping that all would remain quiet on his floor. About 2:30 A.M., Franco was awakened by a loud noise coming from the hall bathroom next to his room. He got up and saw Howell walking down the hall away from the restroom toward his room. His right hand appeared to be bloody. When Franco entered the restroom, he observed that someone had broken the mirror and had thrown a trash can through the restroom window. There was blood in the sink and on the floor.

Questions

1. If you were Franco, what would you do? Explain the steps you would follow.

2. Do you believe there is enough evidence to charge Howell with a violation of university policy, knowing that if you do, Howell might hold it against you and try to get even?

3. Is there anything that could be done to address the "Viking" reputation Howell has developed on the floor and which is encouraged by the residents?

4. What are the advantages and disadvantages of approaching Howell about the damage the night it happened?

Catch Me If You Can

Shirley and Laverne are first semester freshmen. They went to an inner-city school and have not tried to make friends with any of the other women in the living unit. They keep to themselves and have expressed no interest in interacting with the other residents on the floor. Most of the other residents find them somewhat annoying. They have this habit of turning up their heavy-metal music so loud that it disturbs the whole floor. When the residents ask them to turn it down, they refuse to answer the door, or they would hang up on anyone who calls their room to complain. Phyllis is their RA. She has spoken to them about their stereo on several occasions, and she has referred them to the hall judicial council on one occasion. This referral resulted in a fine and a warning. It also resulted in Laverne and Shirley threatening Phyllis.

Phyllis returned to her room late one evening after studying with some of her friends. When she passed Shirley and Laverne's room, their stereo was blasting. She pounded on the door, identified herself, and after some period of time a man opened the door and asked what she wanted. Phyllis noticed the smell of what she believed was marijuana in the room, a wet towel had been placed under the door, and there was a fan blowing air out of the room. There were several scented candles burning and some incense. There was another man in the room with Shirley and Laverne. Phyllis told the group that their stereo was too loud and that they would need to turn it down. Laverne got up and went to the door and closed it in Phyllis's face. Someone then turned the stereo down to an acceptable level.

Questions

1. What would you do at this point if you were the RA?

2. Is there anything the RA might have done differently either before this incident, or during the incident?

3. Two of Phyllis's other residents were standing in the hallway during the incident and saw the whole thing. What do you think will happen if Phyllis decides to ignore the incident and talk to the students at some later time?

4. What is your institution's policy about entering students' rooms and searching for drugs when there is reason to believe that students are using marijuana?

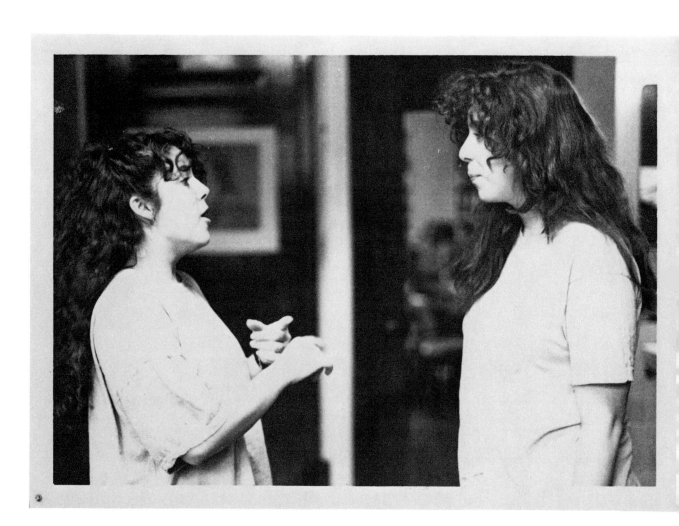

CHAPTER 10

Conflict Resolution

1. A constructive conflict is characterized by what elements? List three.

    1.

    2.

    3.

2. What are the most common causes of conflict?

    1.

    2.

    3.

3. What are the two categories of conflict you are most likely to work with as an RA?

    1.

    2.

4. What are the seven steps Miller and Zoradi identified to manage roommate conflicts?

    1.

    2.

    3.

    4.

5.

6.

7.

5. Give four conflict behaviors which characterize nonconstructive communication in conflict situations and an example of each?

    1.

    2.

    3.

    4.

6. What is meta-communication?

7. Give one technique for preventing threats, coercion, and deception, which sometimes accompanies conflict situations.

Lifestyles of the Rich and Famous

Gloria was a new student at Jones College. She came from a wealthy family in East Texas and was the only child. There was hardly anything that money could buy that her parents did not provide her. She attended Jones College because both her mother and father had attended there. Her mother was on the board of trustees for Jones College, and the family had been financially generous to the College.

Freshman housing was full, and Gloria was assigned a roommate named Amanda. Amanda was also a new freshman. She came from a middle class family. Her mother was a carpenter, and her father taught elementary school. Amanda was attending Jones College with some financial aid, a part-time job in the cafeteria, and help from her parents. She worked throughout high school and was one of four children in the family.

Gloria was not accustomed to taking care of herself. She tended to leave her clothing lying about the room, never made her bed, and left food and other trash about the room. In short, she was a slob. Gloria never had to do these things for herself, and the clutter did not seem to bother her. Periodically, she would gather up her clothes and send them to the cleaners.

In high school Amanda shared a room with her younger sister and was accustomed to keeping her room orderly and to doing a variety of household chores. She was generally a neat person.

The lifestyle differences between the two women extended to other areas. Gloria liked "country and western music"; Amanda liked "rock and roll music." Amanda had to get up early in the morning to work in the cafeteria; Gloria liked to stay up late to watch television and sleep late in the morning.

Gloria did not like sharing a room with another person and was consumed with her own importance. Amanda was not thrilled about living with Gloria, hated how sloppy she was, and secretly wished Gloria would drop out of school. One night after an argument between the two women over Gloria's forgetting to give Amanda a telephone message, Amanda went to the RA and said that she could not stand living with Gloria one more minute. She said that Gloria was a spoiled brat and that if the RA didn't do something about her, she was going to take her softball bat and beat the girl senseless! Not wanting to explain to the President of the College why the daughter of a member of the board of trustees was beaten senseless by her roommate, the RA decided to intercede.

Questions

1. If you were the RA, what steps would you take with Amanda and with Gloria the night that Amanda came to complain?

2. If you were the RA and talked to Gloria and Amanda about their difficulty, what would you do if Gloria stated that she had no interest in resolving the problem and that she would talk with her parents and have Amanda moved to another room?

3. List what you believe to be the major points of disagreement between the two women.

4. What do you think the likelihood is of these two students resolving their lifestyle differences? Should the RA even try to get things worked out between the two women? Why or why not?

5. What is your institution's policy on roommate changes? What would happen if the women could not resolve their problems and neither wished to move?

6. If neither of the women wished to move, who do you think should move and why?

Why Me?

Josh and Stuart were second semester freshmen who were assigned as roommates in the fall semester and became good friends. At their college, fraternity rush is held in the spring semester. Stuart had always wanted to join a fraternity like his older brother and his father. Josh was not sure if he was or was not interested. No one in his family had ever been to college, and Josh was a little concerned whether he could afford the additional cost associated with joining a fraternity. Stuart talked Josh into going through rush with him.

Stuart was particularly interested in the fraternity which his father and brother joined, and was invited to pledge this fraternity. He gladly accepted. Both Stuart and Josh were upset when the same fraternity did not offer Josh the opportunity to pledge. A less prestigious fraternity offered Josh a bid, but he did not know anyone in that fraternity, and with the added cost, he just was not interested.

The relationship between the two boys changed after rush. Stuart spent all of his free time with his pledge brothers and never seemed to have enough time for Josh. Even when Stuart came back to the residence hall room, he usually came with one or two of his friends from the fraternity, and they would spend time in the room talking about things related to the fraternity or people that Josh did not know.

One night about 2:00 A.M., the RA was awakened by loud noises in the hallway. When he opened the door, he saw Stuart and Josh in a fight wrestling on the ground while several of the residents watched. The RA managed to separate the two. He learned that the fight started when Stuart came back to the room and started to search the room for an item that the fraternity required for a scavenger hunt they organized for the pledges. In the commotion of searching the room and turning on the lights, he awoke Josh. Words were exchanged, followed by pushing, and finally a fight began.

Questions

1. What should the RA have done that evening after he stopped the fight and what should he do to follow-up?

2. What emotional issues do you think Josh is feeling about Stuart's involvement in the fraternity? What emotional issues do you believe that Stuart is feeling about his involvement in the fraternity and his relationship with Josh?

3. Assuming that Stuart continues in the fraternity and Josh is not invited to pledge, what are some of the ways you would suggest as the RA that might help them continue their relationship?

4. What do you see as the advantages and disadvantages of a room change for one or both of the students?

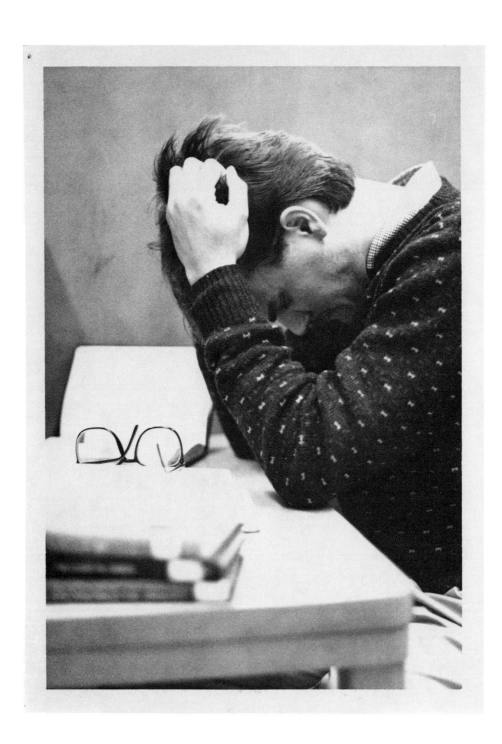

CHAPTER 11

Suicide Intervention

1. Why do many suicides go unreported?

2. Give four theories or causes of suicide.

    1.

    2.

    3.

    4.

3. Give four symptoms of suicide.

    1.

    2.

    3.

    4.

4. One can divide the causes of suicide into two major categories. Identify these two categories.

    1.

    2.

5. State your personal feelings about suicide as it relates to the counseling of students who may be considering it.

6. What is your goal as an RA in counseling a suicidal student?

7. What is the first rule for working with a suicidal student?

8. Give three things that would increase the likelihood of an individual actually attempting suicide.

   1.

   2.

   3.

9. What is a non-suicide contract and how does it work?

10. Many people consider suicide at some time in their life. How do you know when they are serious about it and in danger of doing something about it, and when they are only expressing feelings of depression?

All Alone

Clark and Garrison came to Big East University from California. They had been friends since junior high school and were living as roommates while in college. Garrison started his freshmen year with a full load of classes but began dropping classes about a month into the first semester. By mid-term examinations, he was down to one class. Garrison was a nice young man. He kept to himself, and his only friend on the floor was Clark. Recently, Garrison had started drinking. In high school Garrison would not drink at all, in fact he was involved with a group that worked to keep students from drinking. Garrison's mother and father were divorced. His father was a practicing alcoholic and had been in and out of treatment programs several times. Garrison was not close to his father. His mother was a member of a conservative religious group and was a high school guidance counselor.

Garrison was a very neat and organized person, but recently he had lost interest in keeping things in place. He gave some of his most valuable possessions, including his diary, to Clark. In recent weeks his sleeping had become erratic. He frequently missed class. Garrison started drinking more frequently. Hardly a night went by when he didn't consume eight to ten beers. Sometimes he would sit in his room alone and drink, and other times he would drink with his roommate.

There was one woman who Garrison liked, and he dated her once or twice. She lost interest in him and was now dating someone else in what appeared to be a serious relationship. Garrison felt rejected and somewhat angry over losing out to this other student.

One night Clark returned to his room from the library and found Garrison lying unconscious on the floor of the room. He did not appear to be breathing and could not be awakened. There was a suicide letter written to Clark in his shirt pocket, and the cabinet where Garrison kept medicine and shaving items was open. There was a large bottle of aspirin that was half empty sitting on the sink. The room had a lot of empty cans of beer strewn about the room. Clark ran to get the RA.

Questions

1. Explain your institution's medical emergency procedure for situations such as the one described above.

2. What signs did Garrison give that may have indicated he was suicidal?

3. What is your institution's policy for returning students to school who have attempted suicide?

4. Once the medical personnel arrive to attend to Garrison, what should the RA do to help Clark?

5. What information and assistance can the RA provide to help the medical personnel and the campus police?

6. Should the RA explain what happened to the other students living on the floor? If yes, why and how could this be used educationally? If no, why not and how would you respond to the inquiries from those who observed all the activity on the floor?

Quiet Desperation

Shara had broken up with a young man she dated for about three months. The relationship was over, and she really did not want to see him anymore. It was a difficult relationship for her. She liked the young man but had a difficult time handling the fact that he was African American and she was white. They had unprotected intercourse several times during their relationship. Although Shara's periods were not regular, she thought she had had intercourse only during the times when she was not ovulating.

Shara missed her last period but convinced herself that the stress of breaking up with this young man and her school work were the cause. When she missed her second period, she became concerned. On the chance she was pregnant, she went to a local drug store and bought a home pregnancy test. She took the test, and it was positive for pregnancy. She took the test two more times, and each time it was positive for pregnancy.

She did not want anyone to know about this, least of all her parents who were strong Catholics and had negative attitudes about African Americans. She thought about going to the student health center but ruled it out for fear that her parents might be informed or that they would keep some record of her medical condition. Abortion was an option she considered, but she did not have the money and had been raised to believe that abortion was killing.

Shara was depressed and often cried for no apparent reason. She stopped socializing with the other women on the floor, stopped eating, and slept at least ten to twelve hours a day. Within the past two days, Shara's disposition seemed to improve. She cleaned her room, straightened all of her belongings, and was giving away her favorite pieces of jewelry and her favorite compact disks to her roommate and one other woman on the floor. Her roommate went to the RA, concerned after discovering a used home pregnancy test kit in the room. When she asked Shara if it was hers, Shara said she had never seen it before.

Questions

1. What signs has Shara given that she might be considering suicide?

2. What action would you take if you were Shara's RA? How could the RA help Shara get counseling?

3. What would you do as the RA if Shara denies everything and refuses to go for counseling?

4. What policy does your institution have about informing parents about the confidentiality of student records in the student health center?

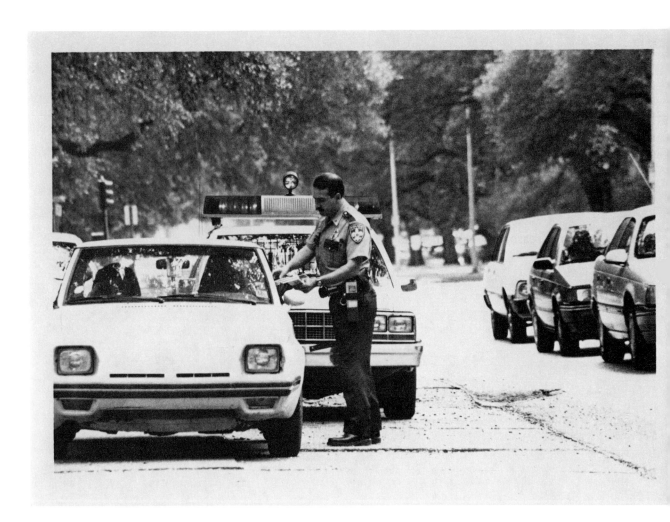

CHAPTER 12

Crime and Victimization in Residence Halls

1. Give three explanations for why men beat women.

    1.

    2.

    3.

2. Give three reasons why women stay in relationships with men who beat them.

    1.

    2.

    3.

3. What are the two most important roles an RA can serve in helping a woman who has been beaten?

    1.

    2.

4. Although a rapist can be any age, the most likely age range for a rapist is?

5. It has been said that rape is not for the sexual gratification of the rapist. If this is true, what does appear to be the motivation?

6. There are two major stages in reaction to rape. What are they, and what are two characteristics of each?

    1.

    2.

7. Give three ways a woman can reduce the risk of rape from a stranger?

    1.

    2.

    3.

8. Give three ways a woman can reduce the risk of an acquaintance or "date" rape?

   1.

   2.

   3.

9. Briefly explain two of the theories about the causes of "date rape".

   1.

   2.

10. What things need to be communicated to men to educate them about "date rape"?

11. What is your institution's procedure for responding to a victim of a rape?

12. What can the RA do to help a woman who has been raped and returns to the residence hall after seeing the police and appropriate medical personnel?

13. List four things that could be done in your residence hall to make it safer for students.

    1.

    2.

    3.

    4.

14. What does the National Crime Prevention Council suggest people do if someone tries to rob them with a weapon?

15. Give four ways an RA can help to make residence halls safer.

    1.

    2.

    3.

    4.

Loving and Fighting

Louis is a senior and has been dating Robin for almost three years. They plan to get married when they graduate. One night the RA is called to Louis's room by several of the men on the floor. When the RA arrives, Louis is in a rage. He is throwing his belongings against the wall and pounding his fist against the wall.

The RA goes into Louis's room and closes the door behind him. He asks Louis "What's wrong?" Louis pauses, regains his composure and tells the RA that he and Robin are having problems. They had a big fight. He shows the RA where Robin scratched him on the arms and face. "You can't let women get away with that kind of thing. Give them an inch and they will take a mile. Unless you keep them in their place they will walk all over you," Louis tells the RA.

The RA asks Louis if he hit Robin. Louis says, "Yes, but only to defend myself, and then only enough times to teach her not to do it again."

The next afternoon the RA sees Louis and Robin together in the dining hall. He notices that she has a bruise on her face. That evening after staff meeting, Louis's RA mentions to Robin's RA that Louis and Robin seemed to have gotten everything worked out. Robin's RA was not aware there was any problem. She had seen the bruise on Robin's face and was told by Robin that it happened playing field hockey with some of her friends.

Questions

1. Is there anything that Robin's RA could say or do to pursue this matter with Robin? If so what?

2. Is there anything that Louis's RA could say or do to pursue this matter with Louis? If so, what?

3. Some people might argue that this is a problem between Robin and Louis and the RAs should not get involved. Do you agree? Why or why not?

4. Give three reasons why Robin may have chosen not to tell anyone about the physical fight she had with Louis.

   1.

   2.

   3.

5. Write an ending to this case study: the best case scenario, and the worst case scenario. Explain which one you think is most likely, and why.

Without Permission

Helen met Patrick at a floor party. Her roommate, Cindy, introduced him to her. Patrick was a resident on the same floor that Cindy's boyfriend was the RA. Patrick and Helen had a nice time on their first date. Patrick was a perfect gentleman on the date and asked permission to kiss her good-night—she consented. On their second date, Patrick took her to dinner, then to a movie. They kissed a few times in his car.

On their third date, Patrick took Helen to an off-campus party where they both had plenty to drink. They went to Patrick's room to listen to music. They started kissing. One thing led to another, and they had intercourse. Helen liked Patrick and did not object. The next morning she felt guilty about having had intercourse with Patrick. She decided that had she not been drinking, she probably would not have had sex with him.

During the week that followed, Helen and Patrick saw each other only once over dinner in the cafeteria. They made plans to go out Friday night to a party at Patrick's fraternity. On Friday, they went to the party. Patrick was drinking, but Helen chose not to. About 11:30 P.M., Patrick asked Helen if she wanted to go upstairs with him to see one of his friend's rooms who was gone for the week-end. She agreed. When they got to the room, Patrick told her that his friend was gone for the whole week-end, and they could have the room all to themselves. He turned on some music and sat next to her on the bed. They started kissing, but when Patrick started to remove Helen's blouse, she said no. Patrick was persistent and managed to remove some of her clothing. When he continued, she again said NO! But, he wouldn't listen. She struggled, but he was much stronger than she. They had intercourse, without her consent. When it was over she began to cry, and asked to be taken home. Patrick tried to calm her down, but Helen didn't want to talk. She just wanted to be taken home.

Patrick drove her to her residence hall. She got out of the car and, without saying another word, walked into her residence hall. She went to her room, changed clothes and took a shower.

On Sunday night, Helen's roommate returned from the weekend. Helen was still upset. She started crying. She told her roommate what happened. Her roommate goes to the RA and has her come to the room. Helen tells the RA what happened, but won't give the RA Patrick's name and does not want the RA to report this to anyone.

Questions

1. Did Patrick have the right to expect that if Helen consented to have intercourse with him that they would continue to have intercourse when they dated? Why or why not?

2. What situational variables in this case study contributed to this act of non-consensual intercourse?

3. Would you describe this act of non-consensual intercourse as "rape"? Why or why not?

4. What are three reasons why Helen might be reluctant to report this assault? Do you think she should? Why or why not?

5. Do you think that Patrick should be criminally prosecuted and/or expelled permanently from the College for his actions as described in the case study? Why or why not?

6. What are the RA's options at this point, and what would you do if you were the RA?

7. Helen's roommate knows that Patrick is responsible for what happened. She tells her boyfriend, who is Patrick's RA. Although, there is no "official" complaint from Helen, what could Patrick's RA do, if anything, to address Patrick's behavior?

8. If Helen would have claimed that Patrick raped her on their third date (the first time they had intercourse) would you agree? Why or why not?

Information on Contemporary Social Issues Confronting College Students

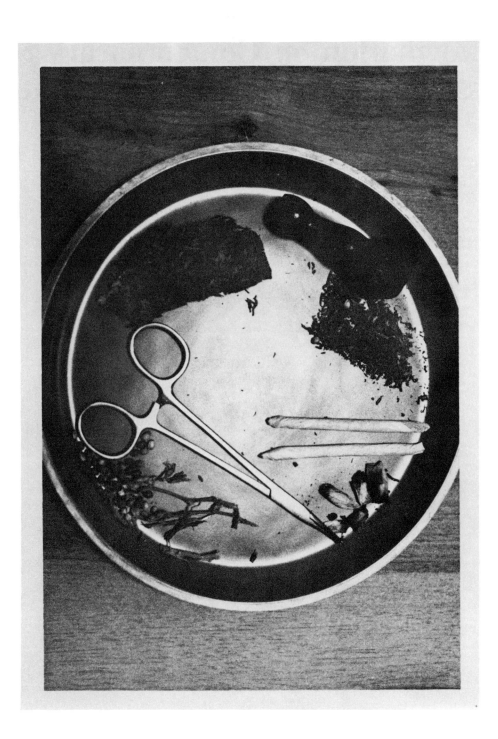

CHAPTER 13

Substance Abuse

1. What are three dangers associated with the use of marijuana?

    1.

    2.

    3.

2. What is the difference in the effect of marijuana and hashish on a person?

3. What is THC?

4. What are two of the harms associated with the use of LSD?

    1.

    2.

5. What is the biggest harm a person faces when he or she buys drugs off the street?

6. What are two of the problems associated with imitation drugs?

    1.

    2.

7. What are two of the problems associated with having drugs in the residence halls?

    1.

    2.

8. What types of drugs are least likely to be detected by RAs and why?

9. What is your institution's procedure for the RA detecting and enforcing campus drug policies?

10. If you encounter someone who has used an hallucinogenic drug (LSD), and is "tripping," what is your institution's policy regarding how you should proceed?

Alcohol Information Quiz

Answer true or false to each of the following questions by circling either T (true) or F (false).

T or F 1. A cold shower and a cup of black coffee will help a person sober up faster.

T or F 2. One beer contains as much alcohol as a jigger (1=4 oz.) of 80-proof whiskey.

T or F 3. The use of alcohol increases sexual ability.

T or F 4. A person will get intoxicated faster by switching drinks rather than by taking the same amount of alcohol in only one form, such as scotch.

T or F 5. About 80 percent of college students use alcohol regularly.

T or F 6. There is a higher percentage of students using alcohol today than there was ten years ago.

T or F 7. The best way to handle someone who is drunk is to be assertive and understanding.

T or F 8. The majority of serious behavioral infractions in residence halls are related to behavior resulting from an excessive use of alcohol.

T or F 9. A student with a drinking problem should be held accountable for his or her actions and made to suffer any consequences.

T or F 10. Most students, by the time they reach college, have made a decision about whether or not to drink.

T or F 11. Eating some butter or drinking a glass of milk will coat your stomach and enable you to drink more.

T or F 12. Having several good drinks before you go to sleep will insure a deep restful sleep.

T or F 13. Vitamins, and/or "the hair of the dog" (small quantity of the alcoholic beverage that was used to become intoxicated) will help a hang-over.

T or F 14. Drinking alcohol will kill brain cells.

T or F 15. Approximately one-third of the students on your floor will have some problem associated with drinking during the coming academic year.

T or F 16. You can die from drinking too much alcohol.

T or F 17. Drinking alcohol in moderate amounts, for most people, does the body little permanent harm.

T or F 18. Blackouts are common after a few drinks.

Winning Through Fear and Intimidation

Dewey's new roommate was not what he expected. He was assigned to live with Allen, a twenty-year-old sophomore from a large urban area near the university. Dewey came to the RA about the third week of school frightened. He told the RA that he needed to tell him something, but he made the RA swear that he wouldn't tell another person.

Dewey believed that Allen was dealing drugs. He had seen some blotter paper cut into squares and some kind of pills which Allen kept hidden inside a broken clock radio next to his bed. Several times Dewey took telephone messages for Allen which sounded suspicious, and there were people he had never seen before coming by the room at odd hours of the day and night.

When Dewey asked Allen what was going on, Allen told him that if he knew what was good for him he would mind his own business and keep his mouth shut. Allen then told Dewey a story about a fellow from Allen's neighborhood who got too nosy and had a terrible accident from which he died. The message Dewey got was clear. He was frightened and believed that Allen had both the means and the disposition to hurt him or anyone else that interfered with his activities.

Dewey told the RA that he thinks that Allen uses some of the drugs regularly himself and is a violent person. Allen has indicated that he does not like the RA and suggested that he might have someone teach the RA a lesson.

Questions

1. Having given his word not to tell anyone, what should the RA do now with the information he has?

2. What dangers does the presence of Allen present to himself and to the other residents of the building?

3. Assuming that Dewey refuses to tell anyone else about this and refuses to talk with the police for fear of reprisal from Allen, what steps can the RA take to help Dewey?

4. Now that the RA has this information about Allen, are there any signs that the RA can look for which might give him enough evidence to pursue this problem independent of the information he has received from Dewey?

5. Write two endings to the above case. One should describe the best outcome for Dewey and Allen, and one should describe, based on your experience, what you think is the most likely outcome.

Let the Good Times Roll

Stacy is 21 years old and is the oldest woman on the floor. She is a sophomore and has a single room. Recently she joined a "little sister" group affiliated with one of the campus fraternities. Since that time her social life has become much more active. At least four nights a week she is out at one of the local college bars or at some party off-campus. The RA has seen her several times come in late at night staggering drunk. One night the RA found her in the restroom vomiting and drunk, and one night she got a call from the RA on duty who asked her to help Stacy to her room because she was too drunk to get there herself. Other residents have told the RA that Stacy often spends the night away from the residence hall.

The hall director received a call from the Dean of Students Office reporting that Stacy has been missing classes. The hall director asked the RA to talk with Stacy about missing classes. The RA found Stacy in her room watching television and drinking something the RA suspected was alcohol. She asked Stacy about her classes and told Stacy that she is concerned about her drinking and her very active social life. Stacy's reaction was unexpected. She became angry and told the RA to mind her own business. She told the RA she will drink as much as she wants when she wants, and she will sleep with whomever she wants when she wants. She told the RA to leave her alone and get out of her room.

Questions

1. What, if anything, can be done to help Stacy?

2. What is your institution's policy about the possession and consumption of alcohol in the residence hall? Do you agree with it? Why or why not? If you do not agree with it, what justification would you give to your residents for enforcing the policy?

3. Stacy believes she has the right to live her life the way she wants, and no one has the right to interfere with her. Do you agree or disagree with Stacy, why or why not?

4. What signs is Stacy giving which indicate that she is experiencing a problem with alcohol?

5. Speculate on some of the reasons for Stacy getting so angry with the RA when the RA expressed concern about her behavior.

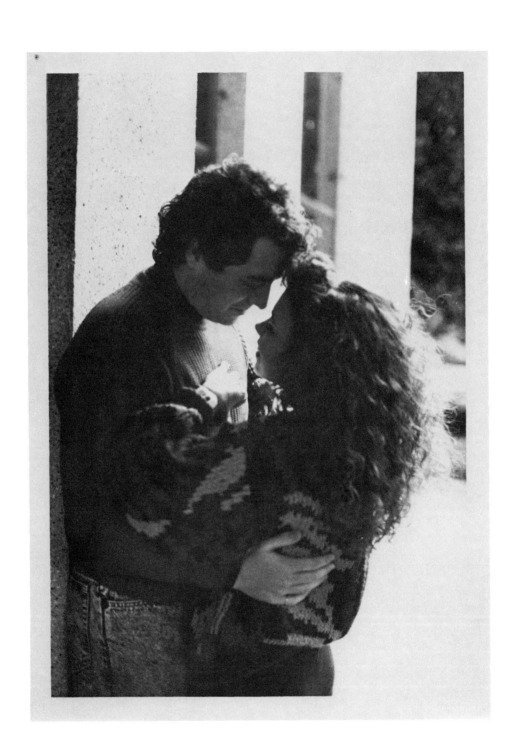

CHAPTER 14

Sexuality

1. Is there a student health center on your campus? If so, what services are offered through the student health center?

2. Can students receive contraceptives at the health center and/or get counseling about sexually transmitted diseases?

3. Is there a family planning or Planned Parenthood clinic near the campus? If so, do they do anonymous HIV testing? If not, where can a student go to get an anonymous HIV test?

4. Is there a Gay Rights Student Organization on your campus? If so, how can a student join the organization?

5. Is there a telephone number that students can call in your community and receive information anonymously about AIDS? About homosexuality? About STD's? About abortions? If so, what are these telephone numbers?

6. Over twenty percent of college women become pregnant during their college career. Most college couples are sexuality active for nine months before they begin using contraceptives. Why is this, and what can be done to get sexually active students who do not want to have children to use birth control?

7. What are the three best methods of contraception after abstinence and sterilization? Give one advantage and one disadvantage of each.

   1.

   2.

   3.

8. What are the three least effective methods of birth control?

   1.

   2.

   3.

9. What are the most common signs of pregnancy?

10. What are some of the ways an RA can help a student after she has had an abortion?

11. What do the anagram AIDS and ARC mean? Give four ways a sexually active person can limit his or her exposure to AIDS.

    1.

    2.

    3.

    4.

12. What is your health center's policy about confidentiality of student medical problems?

13. What is your institution's policy about students who have AIDS and who wish to live in the residence halls?

The Most Difficult Decision of Their Lives

Brenda and Robert have been dating since high school and have talked about getting married when they graduate. Both are sophomores in college. They have been having intercourse throughout most of their relationship but have not regularly used birth control. Brenda does not want anyone to know that she and Robert are having intercourse and will not go to the health center to talk with a physician about birth control pills, an IUD, a diaphragm, or any other method. Brenda has suggested to Robert that he use condoms, but Robert prefers not to. He claims using a condom is too artificial and isn't how "real men" have sex. Most of the time, Robert and Brenda use a combination of the rhythm method and withdrawal.

Brenda has occasionally missed a period, and she was not overly concerned when her period was a week late. She told Robert. He got nervous, and insisted that she take a home pregnancy test. Both were relieved when the test was negative. When she was five weeks late, she got the courage to go to the student health center. The pregnancy test and the gynecological examination showed that she was approximately two months pregnant.

Brenda returns to her residence hall room and, in a state of near hysteria, tells everything to her roommate, who goes to get the RA. When the RA comes into the room, Brenda is sobbing uncontrollably. She tells the RA everything. Brenda does not want the child. She wants to finish college and go to medical school. If she has a baby, she believes this will not be possible. She does not want either Robert or her parents to know that she is pregnant. Robert tends to hold somewhat traditional views, and if Robert finds out, Brenda fears that he will insist on them getting married and keeping the child. She does not want this. Brenda is not sure how her parents would act if they found out, but she is not interested in knowing. She has enough money saved to get an abortion, and that is what she wants to do.

Questions

1. If you were Brenda's RA how would you assist Brenda during this crisis?

2. What are your personal opinions about abortion?

3. Do you think that Robert should be told? Why or why not?

4. Do you think Brenda should tell her parents? Why or why not?

5. If Brenda elects not to tell Robert or her parents, do you think that the university should inform the parents and/or Robert? Why or why not?

6. Brenda's roommate does not want Brenda to have an abortion, and secretly tells Robert. One of Robert's best friends on the floor is the RA, and he goes to his RA to talk about the issue. If you were Robert's RA, how would you help Robert deal with this situation?

Sexual Responsibility

Tony transferred to Farm State University from a community college in New York City. He was a couple of years older than most of the other men in the living unit and was much more worldly. He was very at ease with women and frequently had women in his room for the evening. Tony did not believe in dating just one woman at a time; instead he was interested in "playing the field." He took some pride in the number of sexual conquests he made. Tony was not satisfied with just single encounters but was known to participate in group sexual encounters in his room with other couples on several occasions.

The RA was somewhat befuddled by all of Tony's activity, even though it did not violate any of the University's policies. The RA talked with Tony generally about his activity, particularly about the issue of sexually transmitted diseases. Tony assured him that he knew all about those issues and the RA need not worry.

In time, Tony and the RA became friends. On one or two occasions he got the RA a date with a woman he had previously dated, and the RA had intercourse with her. During the second semester, Tony got what he thought was the flu. It did not seem to go away, and he went to the student health center. Tony tested positive for HIV. When he learned of this, he went to his friend the RA and told him about the test results. He cried and told the RA he was afraid of dying.

When Tony's physical symptoms subsided, he started dating again. He told his friend the RA that he would be "safe" when having sex with others but was not about to give up sex. He would continue to have sex with whomever he wished and figured that, if someone else contacted the disease, that was fate. He got it from someone, and, if he gave it to someone, well that was just their tough luck.

Questions

1. What could the RA do, if anything, to help protect other students from Tony?

2. Should the RA tell his hall director or other University official about Tony? Why or why not?

3. If you were Tony's RA, would you go and have an HIV test? Why or why not?

4. Does the RA have a duty to inform Tony's roommate and the other students in the living unit about Tony testing positive for HIV? Why or why not?

5. Are the other people in Tony's living unit, none of whom he is having sex with, at risk from acquiring AIDS by Tony's presence on the floor? Why or why not?

6. Do you believe that it is possible for Tony to conduct his sex life in such a way that he will not put other people at risk? Why or why not?

7. Do you believe that Tony has a duty to give University health center officials the names of the other students with whom he has had intercourse so that they might be tested for AIDS? If Tony refuses to cooperate, do you believe the University should take steps to remove Tony from the University? Why or why not?

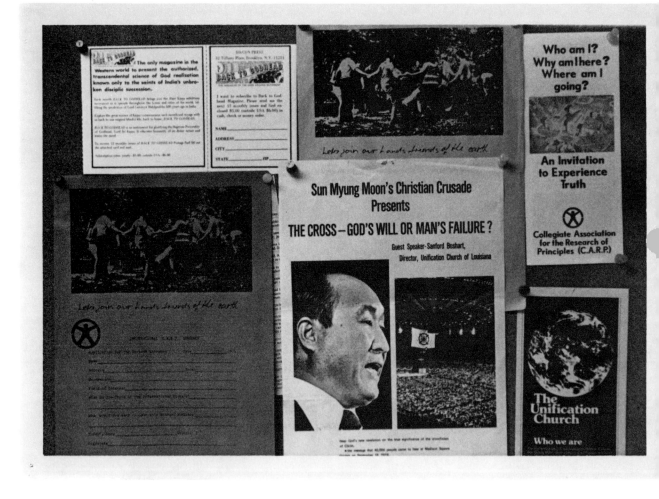

CHAPTER 15

Cult Activities on College Campuses

1. What are three of the distinguishing characteristics of a religious cult?

    1.

    2.

    3.

2. There are three general phases to the conversion process. What are they?

    1.

    2.

    3.

3. Why are college students particularly susceptible to recruitment by cults?

4. Give three reasons why a student might join a religious cult?

    1.

    2.

    3.

5. What are three harms to the individual associated with involvement in a cult?

    1.

    2.

    3.

6. Give four things that you can observe in students which might indicate that they are becoming involved in a cult?

    1.

    2.

    3.

    4.

7. If a student joins a cult, what do you believe the RA or the university can or should do about it?

8. Give four ways in which the RA can assist students in protecting themselves from cult groups?

   1.

   2.

   3.

   4.

9. Explain how cult groups deceive students into joining their group.

10. What is meant by the Lifton's term ''milieu control,'' and how is it used to influence a person's decision to join a cult?

In Search of Spiritual Fulfillment

Ever since Gilbert moved into the living unit as a new freshmen, he has acted a bit strange. He never seemed to fit in with the other residents. He kept to himself and was known as a loner. Recently, the RA noticed that he always seemed to be dressed in black and had become infatuated with silver jewelry. He started wearing an inverted silver cross in one ear, and had etched with pen the numbers "666" into his forearm. He decorated his room with posters from heavy-metal music groups. His collection of recent recreational reading concerned the occult, witchcraft, and Satanism.

Gilbert would often spend the weekend off-campus. One Sunday Gilbert returned to the residence hall exhausted and appeared to be intoxicated. Gilbert's roommate came to get the RA when he found Gilbert in the hall shower crying.

Gilbert told the RA that he was initiated into a group called the Disciples of Natas. He was crying because he finally had a group who accepted him and because he would be leaving college for awhile to live on a farm outside of town where he would be trained by one of the disciples in the ways of the group. He said he would be allowed to attend classes and was just going to move out of the residence hall until his training was complete. He was to pack his personal belongings to be ready to leave the residence hall that night at midnight. He was forbidden to say anything else about the group, where the farm was located, or who was to meet him. This information was all to be kept secret, and Gilbert had taken a blood oath to not reveal anything else about the group.

Questions

1. Gilbert is over the age of eighteen and as a adult has the right to come and go from the residence hall at his discretion. What if anything should the RA do?

2. Give three early warning signs that might have indicated that Gilbert was susceptible to the influence of a cult group?

   1.

   2.

   3.

3. Do you believe that the RA might have been able to do anything to help Gilbert avoid this group or groups like this? If so what?

4. The group with which Gilbert has associated himself is obviously a Satanic group. Would your attitude toward Gilbert's participation be different if the group was a ''Born Again Christian'' group? Why or why not?

The Seeker

Ginger is an RA in a large coed residence hall at Small State College. Recently Ginger has noticed posters in her hall asking students to attend a free lecture on world justice and hunger. It is sponsored by a group that is on the Dean of Students "Recognized Student Organizations" list. The group calls itself the "World League of Justice." One of Ginger's residents, Carmen, went to several meetings about the group and has invited a representative from the organization to meet with about a dozen or so of her friends in the floor lounge to learn more about the organization. Carmen has put some posters on the hall bulletin board and her door inviting anyone interested in world justice to come to the meeting.

Ginger decides to attend the meeting. The representative from the World League of Justice is well prepared. He is dressed in a white shirt and tie and is accompanied by an older man who is dressed similarly. They show a film about the organization, distribute some literature and serve some refreshments. The program is wonderful. Almost everyone was crying by the end of the film, and most felt a little guilty for having so much while others had so little.

The speakers invited everyone to a two day workshop at the organization's convention center located in a community about a three hour drive from the campus. There the students will be introduced to the movement for world justice and learn how to get in touch with their own natural commitment to share and give to others. A "bus ticket" is distributed to anyone who might be interested, and a roster of interested people is passed around the room. A special bus will stop by the residence hall early Saturday morning to collect all of those willing to help others less fortunate than themselves.

Several of the people on the floor receive a telephone call from the speaker reminding them about the workshop and getting a confirmation on workshop attendance. Ginger finds a flyer under her door from the organization reminding her about the workshop and again inviting her to attend the two day retreat.

Questions

1. What are some of the signs that this group may be a cult?

2. What is your institution's policy for recognition of student organizations?

3. Is there a difference between a registered student organization and a recognized student organization at your institution? If so what is it?

4. Does recognition or registration of a student organization with your institution imply that your institution endorses the philosophy or programs of that organization? Why or why not?

5. What is your institution's policy on door to door solicitation for religious purposes, for organizational purposes, or for commercial purposes?

6. What should the RA do following the presentation by this organization to help her residents make an informed decision about the activities of this group?

7. If College officials do not have any concrete evidence that the organization is a cult, do you think they have any responsibility to parents to inform them of this activity?

8. Do you believe that Colleges and Universities should deny recognition or registration to student groups who are associated with cult-type organizations? Why or why not?

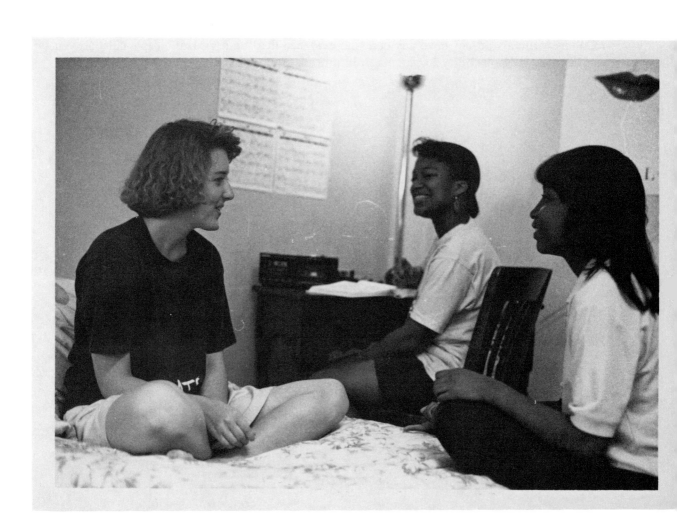

CHAPTER 16

Culture Diversity: Race, Gender, and Sexual Orientation

1. What are stereotypes, and how do they help us in perceiving the world around us?

2. What is the difference between prejudice and discrimination?

3. Briefly describe three sources of prejudice.

    1.

    2.

    3.

4. Give three reasons why people of color often feel unwelcome at predominantly white universities?

    1.

    2.

    3.

5. What is "cross-cultural communication," and how can the RA improve it among the residents in his or her living unit?

6. How does the socialization process for women in college influence the nature and complexity of their relationships with others?

7. What is sexual harassment?

8. Does your institution have a policy on sexual harassment? If so, briefly explain the policy?

9. Give three reasons given for explaining why people are homosexual and tell which one you find most plausible and why?

    1.

    2.

    3.

10. What is "homophobia" and why are young men more likely to be homophobic than women or older men?

11. Identify two problems a homosexual male is likely to experience in a men's residence hall and give two ways his RA could help.

    1.

    2.

Ways to help
  1.

  2.

  3.

13. If the hall director or other university official has knowledge that a student is homosexual, do you think that this information should be shared with the RA? Why or why not?

14. What is your institution's policy for making roommate changes when the request is based on dissatisfaction with the other person's race? What is your institution's policy for making roommate changes when the request is based on dissatisfaction with the other person's sexual orientation?

Race:

Sexual Orientation:

Cross-Cultural Miscommunication

Scott always wanted to attend Big Sky University and was thrilled when he was granted admission. He moved into his residence hall on the first day the halls opened and was primed for what he envisioned would be the ultimate in the college experience. He did not have a roommate and was eager to meet the person who he hoped would become one of his closest friends.

When Scott returned from playing a pick-up game of basketball, he discovered three large suitcases in his room belonging to what was obviously going to be his roommate. He waited in his room for almost two hours before a young man entered and introduced himself as Mohamid. The man proceeded to tell Scott that he was twenty-one and a citizen of Iran. He came to the United States on a scholarship from his government to study engineering. He had been married since he was eighteen. His plans were to study alone in the United States for a year, return home and bring his wife to live with him in the United States while he finished his studies.

Mohamid was a strict Moslem. He prayed five times a day, observed all of the Moslem holidays, and read the Koran each day. His English was understandable, if you listened carefully, but he often had difficulty.

Scott did not know what to do. This was not the roommate Scott had envisioned he would have. He was from a small town and didn't know any international students. The only thing he knew about Iran was from the television news media. Much of what they reported about the political climate of the country was unfavorable. Scott did not want to cause any trouble and was not sure what he could do about it. Mohamid had made friends with some other Iranian students and, when Scott returned to his room the next day, his roommate had three other Arab students in the room, speaking Arabic. Scott didn't know what to do, where to sit, or how to fit in with these other men.

By the time classes started, Scott just couldn't deal with his disappointment and frustration any longer. He wanted a roommate who was like himself and who had the same interests. He went to the RA and asked him to please help him get a room change. The residence halls at Big Sky University were full, and no roommate changes were allowed for four weeks, after which time room changes would be honored to fill unclaimed room reservations and vacancies created by those students who chose not to stay. The room change requests would be honored on a class priority system beginning with seniors. There were always more requests than could be accommodated both for roommate changes and from students who at the last minute decided they wanted to live in the halls but didn't reserve a room. The one exception to the four-week waiting period and priority system was a "special situation petition" supported by the RA and the hall director.

Scott asked to be granted a "special situation petition." He wrote the following:

Dear Director of Residence Life:

I need a room change. My roommate is not what I expected. He doesn't talk English and he is married. He is always bringing his friends into the room, and they talk in Arabic. I can't understand them.

Once I walked in on all of them praying together on the floor. I didn't know what to do, and they got angry when I came in and got my books.

I need to get out of this room. This isn't what I thought Big Sky University was supposed to be like. I want a roommate that I can do stuff with. I talked this over with my Mom and Dad, and they want me to move too. If you want, you can call them.
Very truly yours,
Scott

P.S. If I don't get moved, I might have to drop-out of college.

Questions

1. If you are Scott's RA, would you support his "special situation petition" to move within the first four-week period? If not during the first four week period, would you support his request for special consideration after the four-week period? Explain your answer.

2. Is there anything the RA might be able to do to ease Scott's concerns?

3. If Mohamid was an African American student, born and raised in the United States, and his friends were African American students, would you feel differently about Scott, a white student, requesting special consideration for a room change? Explain your answer.

4. What are the three largest racial groups on your campus and what are the complaints students give when they do not want to live with a member of one of these groups?

    1.

    2.

    3.

5. Some institutions have adopted a policy that forbids roommate changes on the basis of race, creed, color, national origin, disability, or sexual orientation. What is your opinion of such a policy?

Close Friends

Seymour was starting his second year at State University. He was a good student. His overall grade point average was over 3.5 (A = 4.0). He studied hard and wanted to get into a good medical school when he finished. This was also his second year in the same residence hall on the same floor. He returned to live in the hall because it was simpler than finding a new place, and he knew most of the men with whom he would be living. One of the things that Seymour liked about his floor was that it was a study floor. Quiet hours were strictly enforced after 7:00 p.m. each school night. This gave him the time he needed to study.

Seymour had requested a single room, but none were available. The roommate assigned to live with him was a freshman named Mike. Seymour had a roommate much like himself last year: a person who studied, kept somewhat to himself, but had a number of friends on the floor. Two things were very noticeable about Mike. First, he was very good looking. He lifted weights regularly and had been a high school varsity athlete. The second noticeable thing about Mike was that he spent a lot of time talking about sex and girls. Seymour was not accustomed to all of this talk about sex and had had only one sexual experience with a girl he dated in high school.

Seymour liked and admired Mike. He found that the more time he spent with Mike the closer they became. Seymour began having sexual fantasies about Mike. The more he thought about it, the more appealing the idea of having sex with another man became. One night he got the courage to go to a local gay bar. There he met another college student who was gay, and Seymour went to this student's apartment where Seymour had sex with another man for the first time in his life. Seymour had really mixed feelings about what had happened. One night when Seymour and Mike were drinking and talking late into the evening, Seymour, who trusted Mike and still harbored sexual feelings for him, told Mike about his one homosexual experience and that he really liked Mike.

Mike was shocked and a little frightened. The conversation ended when Mike changed the subject. About an hour after Seymour went to sleep, Mike left the room and went to the RA's room and awoke him. He told the RA that he had to tell him something in strictest confidence. Mike related everything that Seymour had told him that evening. He also said that, although he liked Seymour, he wasn't about to live with any ''queer'' and that he was afraid Seymour might try to rape him or something. He was also afraid that Seymour might now have AIDS and that he was going to be contaminated. Mike demanded that the RA get rid of Seymour, but he did not want Seymour to know that he told the RA this information, or that he was the one requesting that Seymour be moved. All Mike knew for sure was that he was scared of living with a gay student.

Questions

1. If you were the RA, what would you say to Mike that evening?

2. If you were the RA, what action, if any, would you take with Mike?

3. What action, if any, would you take with Seymour?

4. What developmental crisis is Seymour facing?

5. What developmental crisis is Mike facing?

6. Do you think Seymour is gay? Why or why not?

7. What would you do if you were Mike? Would you have responded similarly?

Harassment

Cranston was a Ph.D. candidate, and as part of his assistantship he agreed to live in the university's "Living and Learning Residence Hall." He lived in a special apartment in the hall reserved for the faculty member in residence and taught one introductory philosophy course in the residence hall. Students in this class lived in the residence hall and were part of the special "Living and Learning" program. The residence hall was coed, and the class of twenty that Cranston taught had ten women in it. Cranston was married and his wife was expecting their first child. She was a line supervisor for a Potato Chip company in the area and worked eight to five, five days a week.

Cranston flirted with all of the women in his class. He liked to start each class with a joke. Most had sexual overtones and generally were degrading to women. Cranston showed particular attention to one female student in the class. Her name was Shawn. She liked the attention she got from Cranston and encouraged it. She would come to class in very seductive clothing and would flirt shamelessly with Cranston whenever she had the opportunity. Time and time again she would invite Cranston to her room to see something in her room, and he would go willingly.

Shawn bragged to her roommate that she wanted to have an affair with Cranston. She was carrying a heavy course load this semester and could not afford to put in as much effort in the philosophy class as Cranston was requiring. She also thought he was cute. So she decided she might be able to get him to give her a break if she were particularly nice to him.

It wasn't long before Cranston and Shawn were involved in a sexual arrangement by mutual consent. About half the time Shawn would go to Cranston's apartment in the residence hall after his wife went to work. The other half of the time, they would go the Shawn's room while Shawn's roommate had class.

Most of the women on Shawn's floor knew or suspected what was going on. At the end of the fall semester, Shawn got her grade for the course. She earned a "C" in the course. She was angry because she expected an "A." Cranston and Shawn had a big fight over the grade, and Shawn went to her RA.

Shawn told her RA that Cranston had slept with her and that she wanted to file sexual harassment charges against him.

Questions

1. Given that Shawn was a willing and consenting participant in the affair, does she have grounds for filling charges of sexual harassment against Cranston? Why or why not?

2. Do the students in Cranston's class have grounds for filling charges of sexual harassment against him? If so what are the grounds?

3. If you were Shawn's RA, how would you advice her on what to do or not do?

4. If Cranston were a bachelor and he had an affair with Shawn, would it make any difference in your feelings about what happened? Explain your answer.

5. If Shawn were a homosexual man and Cranston was bisexual, do you think Shawn would still have grounds for filing sexual harassment charges? Why or why not?

6. Do you see anything wrong with a member of the faculty having an affair with a student who is not in his or her class and is not likely to be at anytime in the future? Why or why not? How does your institution's policy address this issue?

7. If you were the president of the university and this situation came to your attention, what action, if any, would you take against Cranston? What action, if any, would you take against Shawn?

Educational Outreach

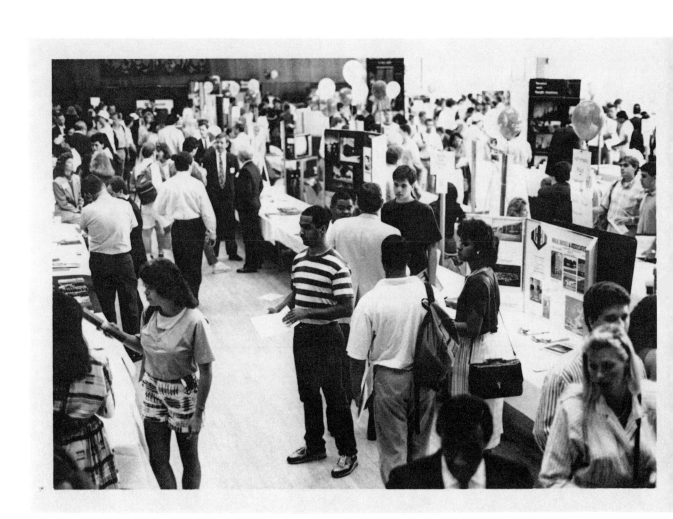

CHAPTER 17

Educational Programming

1. Give four educational reasons for programming in the residence halls.

    1.

    2.

    3.

    4.

2. What are four goals of programming?

    1.

    2.

    3.

    4.

3. Why should programming be established early in the academic year?

4. How do "spontaneous" programs differ from "last-minute" programs?

5. Identify three ways to do a needs assessment for programming in your living unit.

   1.

   2.

   3.

6. Write one performance objective for programming on your floor for next semester.

7. What is the best time to do programming on the floor and why?

8. List two of the best programs you attended in the residence halls and explain what made them good programs.

   1.

   2.

9. Identify a theme for a series of programs (other than movies) which you believe would be of interest to your residents and identify at least three programs, each in a different category of educational program, which would fit within the theme you identified.

10. What programming model, if any, is used at your institution in the residence halls?

Trying to Get by in Programming

Carlo was an RA for the third year. He had lost much of his enthusiasm for the job and had become somewhat cynical in his last year of school. He did not see any reason to inconvenience himself by organizing educational programs on his floor. The problem was that he was required to do at least two programs on his floor each semester. If he failed, the university's policy was to terminate the employment of the RA. All RAs clearly understood this, and it was given to them in writing as part of their contract.

When mid-term examinations were past and he still had not done his first program, the hall director called Carlo into his office for a discussion about the importance of programming. Carlo called a friend of his who was a representative to the student government association to come to his floor and speak. He announced that there was a "required" floor meeting for all of the students on his floor. Carlo's speaker came and talked for ten minutes about SGA and what it does for students and how students could get involved. The speaker then offered to answer questions. No one had any questions, and the meeting was adjourned after a few comments from Carlo about noise on the floor.

As the semester drew to a close, Carlo had not done his second program, and he knew he needed to have one for his hall director. Carlo wrote a programming report that said that members of the floor were organized to attend a sporting event followed by a discussion group about the relationship of college sports to the education of students.

Upon reading this programming report, the hall director approached one of the students on Carlo's floor to inquire about the program. The student did not have any idea what the hall director was talking about. When the hall director quizzed Carlo, he puffed up his explanation but finally admitted that the "program" was nothing more than a group of seven of the men who lived on the floor going to a home football game together and talking about the game afterwards. Anyone from the floor who had tickets was welcome to attend.

Questions

1. If you were Carlo's hall director, would you terminate him for failure to complete two programs as required by his contract? Why or why not?

2. Identify five things that Carlo did not do in his first program, which, had he done, would have made it a better program.

3. If you were Carlo's hall director, and you decided to let Carlo remain an RA, what guidelines would you give him to make sure he did a better job in programming the second semester?

4. If you were Carlo's hall director and wanted to convince Carlo of the need to do educational programs on his floor, what would you tell him?

Program Problem Solver

Dixie was a new RA in an all freshmen residence hall. It was an older hall and had long, double-loaded, single hallways which housed about sixty women; two women were assigned to each room. Dixie wanted to do a good job in her first semester and decided to schedule twice as many programs as was expected. She was well organized and planned all of her programs before the semester started. The six programs she scheduled were (1) a speaker on the student health center services, (2) a movie about birth control, (3) a speaker about the university's honor program, (4) a speaker from the university police office to discuss campus safety, (5) a movie on the history of the university and some of the tourist attractions in the community in which the university was located, and (6) a speaker from the Public Health Department to talk about AIDS.

At the end of the first semester, the Office of Residence Life administers a survey which assesses the social climate of each floor and the social climate of the building. The surveys from Dixie's floor showed that her residents rated the social climate of the living unit low. They felt isolated, were dissatisfied with the experience in the hall, and had no sense of belonging or community.

Questions

1. Give two reasons why you think that students on Dixie's floor may have rated the social climate low.

   1.

   2.

2. Give two strengths and three weaknesses in Dixie's programming.

   Strengths:

      1.

      2.

   Weaknesses:

      1.

      2.

      3.

3. If you were Dixie's hall director, what approach to programming would you suggest that Dixie use to build community on her floor?

4. List three programs which were held on your floor or in your building which you believe helped students develop a sense of community.

    1.

    2.

    3.

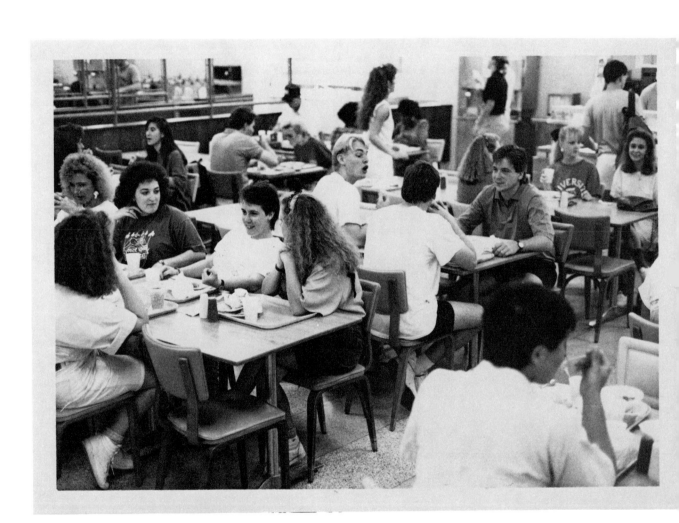

CHAPTER 18

Community Development

1. Write your definition of "community."

2. How can you tell when there is or is not a sense of community on a floor?

3. Why is a sense of community on a residence hall floor important? Give at least three reasons.

   1.

   2.

   3.

4. What are three important elements to establishing a community?

   1.

   2.

   3.

5. Give an example of a program or activity on your floor which helped to make the residents more of a community, and explain why.

6. What role do intramural and other competitive sports play in the establishment of community on a residence hall floor?

7. What are the barriers hall directors face in establishing a sense of community within an entire residence hall?

8. Identify two groups on your campus which you believe have a strong sense of community, and explain why.

    1.

    2.

9. Do you believe students on your campus have a strong sense of identification (or feeling of community) with your institution? Why or why not?

10. Is there any way that the experience of living in a residence hall helps or hinders the process of developing a sense of community with your institution?

11. What role, if any, do rituals and ceremonies play in the establishment of community on your residence hall floor and at your institution?

Altogether

Rita was having a difficult time getting the students on her floor to interact with each other. About 40 women lived on her floor; half were residents last year and half were new freshmen. The returning students were grouped together in three clusters near the hall bathrooms. The new students were scattered about the hall and formed separate little pockets. By the end of the fall semester, Rita had five different groups of eight women each on her floor. All the women seemed reasonably satisfied. There was occasionally some tension between one group of returning students at one end of the hall and some of the new students at the other end of the hall, but it was usually nothing serious.

None of the women on the floor knew all of the other students on the floor. Even Rita had a hard time remembering the names of all of her residents. At the two floor meetings she held in the fall semester, the students were disinterested in having any social functions. Most of the returning women were involved with activities and jobs outside the residence hall, and most of the new students were pledging a sorority and did not have time for any floor functions.

Rita met her programing requirement with two programs: one on sex education and one on drug education. Both were good programs, but poorly attended.

Questions

1. Given the circumstances cited above, how important is it that Rita establish a sense of community among all 40 of her residents?

2. Is it necessary for all 40 of the students in a living unit to be close with one another for there to be a sense of community on the floor? Explain your answer.

3. Is there any way that Rita may have been able to increase the communication and trust between the new students and returning students? Either explain how she could accomplish this or explain why it could not be accomplished.

4. What do you see as the advantages and disadvantages to the development of community when mixing freshmen and upperclass students together in a residence hall?

5. When Rita is evaluated by her hall director, do you think she should receive a low performance rating because she was unable to establish a sense of community among all of her residents?

The War Between the Corridors

Oumar was the RA on the twelfth floor of a sixteen story high rise residence hall. His 40 residents were all freshmen or transfer students. The building was constructed like a "V." He had 20 residents down each corridor, and his room was located at the junction of the two corridors. There were two flag football teams from his floor. One team called themselves 12 North and was composed of the students from the North corridor. The other team called themselves 12 South and was composed of the students from the South corridor.

The teams were in the same intramural league, and one evening after dinner they played a game of flag football. A fight broke out at the game, and both teams were suspended from participation in intramural football for that semester. By the time the students returned to the residence hall, tempers were running high.

Oumar found several students standing in front of the elevator yelling at one another and making threats. During the week that followed, students who were on 12 South had water dumped under their doors twice, glue put in the locks of two of the doors in that corridor, and the restroom at their end of the hall "trashed" with paper and broken beer bottles.

Students on 12 North were not spared destruction. For every act of vandalism that occurred in the South Corridor, there was retaliation. If two door locks were filled with glue in the South corridor, the students from 12 South would see to it that there were at least three filled with glue in the North corridor as retaliation. The fire alarm pull station had been pulled on several occasions at both ends of the floor.

The students from 12 South took to wearing T-shirts that showed a rebel flag inscribed with "12 South." Not to be outdone, the students on 12 North had their own T-shirt designed showing the American flag and bearing the inscription "12 North."

Oumar tried to catch the students responsible by sitting up all night, but was not successful. It was apparent that the whole thing had become a game, and each corridor was out to defeat the other by besting them in acts of vandalism. On two occasions, someone jammed his door shut by placing pennies against the lock so that he could not open the door, and on several occasions water was dumped under his door. Oumar tried to find out who was responsible, but no one would tell him. The only information he would receive was allegations about how one group or the other did this or that. Students on each corridor were very close with the men from their corridor; but, the two groups of students disliked each other, and neither group liked Oumar or the hall director.

Questions

1. If you were Oumar, what would you do to end the conflict and floor vandalism?

2. Identify the elements of community (observable behavior) existing on Oumar's floor?

3. Is there anything that Oumar could have done when the conflict first arose to diffuse the hostility between the two groups? If so, what?

4. The Dean of Students was consulted about the problems on the twelfth floor, and she gave the students until the end of the semester to resolve their differences or she would instruct the Director of Residence Life to disband the entire floor and send each student to a different living unit on campus. What do you see as the advantages and disadvantages of this solution?

5. List at least four programs or activities that Oumar might have done in the first few weeks of school to build community on the floor as a whole.

   1.

   2.

   3.

   4.

6. What are the possible negative repercussions to students from living on a floor characterized by this ongoing conflict?

PART VI

RA Survival Skills

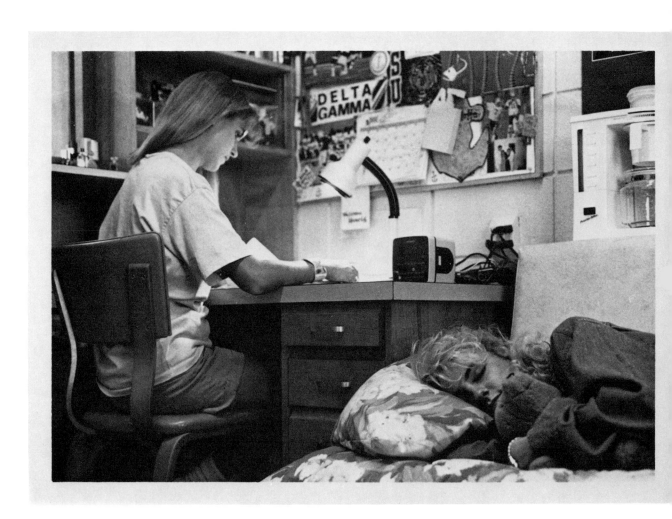

CHAPTER 19

Time Management

1. What is time management?

2. What is the most common mistake people make in managing their time?

3. Time can be categorized into three general categories. What are they?

   1.

   2.

   3.

4. Give two examples of "necessary other imposed time" and two examples of "unnecessary other imposed time."

Necessary:

1.

2.

Unnecessary:

1.

2.

5. Identify two ways to control unnecessary other imposed time.

1.

2.

6. Using the time planning calendar provided in this chapter, identify all of your "predictable time" for the current week.

7. Below identify the things that you need to accomplish for the week. (Note, a "To Do" list should be done each day. A week-long list helps with overall planning, but is subject to change.)

To Do List

1.

2.

3.

4.

5.

6.

7.

8.

9.

10.

11.

12.

8. On your "To do list" above, assign an "A" to those that are most important, a "B" to those which are of secondary importance, and a "C" to those of least importance.

9. Schedule your discretionary time on the planning calendar provided.

10. How much unscheduled time do you have and how much time have you allowed yourself for recreation and relaxation?

11. What can you do to increase your unscheduled time?

Time Planning Calendar

Time	Mon.	Tues.	Wed.	Thur.	Fri.	Sat.	Sun.
7:00 am							
8:00							
9:00							
10:00							
11:00							
12:00 noon							
1:00 pm							
2:00							
3:00							
4:00							
5:00							
6:00							
7:00							
8:00							
9:00							
10:00							
11:00							
12:00 midnight							
1:00 am							
2:00							
3:00							

Hurry, Scurry

Hope was one of the most meticulous people you could meet. She was a master of efficiency and time scheduling. She awoke every morning to an alarm clock and checked her schedule for the day. She would then make a "to do" list outlining everything that she needed to do for the day. Time was precious, and she was a miser with it. She allotted herself exactly twenty minutes in the restroom each morning, twelve minutes to get dressed, ten minutes to get to breakfast, twenty minutes to eat, and fifteen minutes to get to her first class. Her whole day each day was scheduled with the same meticulous care to every minute of every day. Her efficiency was the marvel of everyone.

Hope was an RA and needed to control the time imposed on her from others. To do this, she established one and a half hours a night when she would talk with her residents. There was a sign-up list on the outside of her door and students with a problem could make an appointment to see her by signing their name for a fifteen minute block of time. When the student's fifteen minutes had elapsed, and if there was another student scheduled to see her, she would politely tell the student that her time had expired and she would need to make another appointment if there was more that needed to be said on the topic.

What was surprising about Hope was that she always seemed to be in a rush. She compulsively looked at her wrist watch, and when someone talked with her they would get the feeling that they were keeping her from someplace she needed to be.

Hope met all of the requirements of the Residence Life Office and did not have any more problems on her floor than any of the other RAs in her building.

Questions

1. What are some of the good and bad time management techniques Hope employs?

2. Would you like to be a student on Hope's floor? Why or why not?

3. If you were Hope's hall director, what suggestions would you give her to overcome her compulsion about scheduling?

Happenstance

Albert was a free spirit. He loved the RA job and everything about it. He loved life and lived a carefree, easy-going life style. He laughed at people who were slaves to schedules and liked to let life unfold for him. One of the things that gave Albert joy was playing cards; he was very good at it. Daily he and three other residents played pinochle.

Albert was a great guy. All the men on his floor liked him, and he would always make time for them. Albert had a few problems. One of them was that he was always late to meetings. it was a joke among the staff that staff meeting would start on "AT," which stood for "Albert time." Albert was a pretty good student and did not see any reason to bother attending classes. He had the exam schedule and knew someone in each of his classes who could supply him with class notes.

The new freshmen looked-up to Albert. They all admired his great personality, free life-style, and his ability not to let little things like other people's schedules and time commitments get in the way of what made him feel good.

Questions

1. Does Albert make a good role model for other students on the floor? Why or why not?

2. What do you see as the long range implications of Albert's lack of concern about time management?

3. How does it make you feel when other people keep you waiting, are continually late, or forget commitments?

4. If you were Albert's hall director, how would you address the issue of Albert being late for staff meetings?

5. If you were Albert's hall director, would you take some action to get Albert to attend class and manage his time better, or do you think that this is Albert's business and should not be anyone's concern how he chooses to spend his time?

6. How could the hall director help Albert get control of his time without writing a schedule for him?

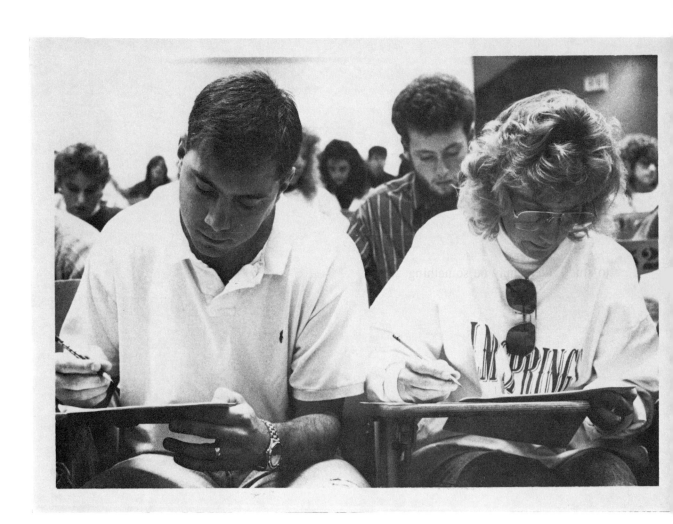

CHAPTER 20

Study Skills

1. In each of the questions below first identify the false assumption(s) that is made and second give a rebuttal to the rationalization.

   EXAMPLE:

   Rationalization: I find it easier to study when I am under pressure. So I will not do any studying until it gets time for a test.

   False Assumption: The greater the pressure the easier it is to study.

   False Assumption: Quality of academic work is related to the degree of pressure to get it done.

   False Assumption: The amount of studying needed to pass a test is proportional to the time between the date of the test and the moment at which the pressure builds to the point which causes the person to study.

   Rebuttal: Studying may seem easier under pressure, but if you wait until the last minute, you may not assemble all of the material you need, you will not have time to rewrite or review some material that you know less well, you may not be able to get all of the materials or notes that you need to study, there may be something unexpected that happens that prevents you from studying, etc.

   a. Rationalization: The world won't come to an end if I put this class project off, so it does not really matter if I delay.

      False Assumption(s):

      Rebuttal:

b. Rationalization: I'll put the project off until I feel like I am in the mood to do it.

False Assumption(s):

Rebuttal:

c. Rationalization: I waited until the last minute to do the term paper the last time and it worked, so why should I not do it the same way again?

False Assumption(s):

Rebuttal:

d. Rationalization: If I wait until the last minute to do this term paper I won't need to spend too much time on it and will save myself time and effort.

False Assumption(s):

Rebuttal:

e. Rationalization: If I do the project now, instead of putting if off until next week, I may never get the same opportunity to enjoy what I am doing right now.

False Assumption(s):

Rebuttal:

f. Rationalization: I would have gotten around to doing the project sooner, but there were circumstances beyond by control that prevented me from doing it.

False Assumption(s):

Rebuttal:

g. Rationalization: No one really cares if I finish the term paper or not. The professor probably won't even read it.

False Assumption(s):

Rebuttal:

h. Rationalization: I should not have to do this homework. It is unfair for the professor to expect me to do all of this work. He/she has unrealistic expectations.

False Assumption(s):

Rebuttal:

i. Rationalization: College is supposed to be more than just studying.

False Assumption(s):

Rebuttal:

j. Rationalization: I have been working hard all quarter and I deserve a break, so I'll work on the project some other time.

False Assumption(s):

Rebuttal:

2. How does the place where one studies influence the process of studying?

3. Describe the ideal study environment for you, and explain why.

4. There are five steps which can be used to study a textbook, what are they?

   1.

   2.

   3.

   4.

   5.

5. How would you define "good note taking" in class?

6. Why is tape recording a class lecture a less effective studying method than note taking?

7. Identify the four principal ways people employ to master information?

1.

2.

3.

4.

8. Give two suggestions for taking an essay exam?

1.

2.

9. What is test anxiety, and what are some ways it can be controlled?

10. What is your institution's policy on academic dishonesty, and what is the most likely penalty a student would receive for academic dishonesty at your institution?

Elroy

Elroy is a first quarter freshman. He was an average student in high school partially because he seldom studied. When he arrived at the university, he moved into a residence hall. He and his roommate both went through fraternity rush and both pledged the prestigious XX fraternity. Elroy is very excited about becoming part of the fraternity and has devoted much of his time to making sure he knows all of the actives, attends all of the social functions and intramural athletic events in which the fraternity is involved. When Elroy pledged the fraternity, he was told that the national fraternity regulations require a pledge to have a minimum grade point average of at least a 2.0 (on a scale of 4.0 = A) and to be a full-time student carrying not less than 15 quarter hours in the quarter prior to initiation. It is now the fifth week of the ten week quarter and Elroy realizes that he is not doing very well in the five three-hour classes he is taking as a new freshman.

Elroy is not the only one to notice that he is not studying. The RA also notices Elroy is not studying and goes to talk with him. The conversation goes like this:

RA: Elroy, what classes are you taking this quarter and how are you doing in your classes?

Elroy: All right—not great. I am carrying five three-hour courses: English 101, Math 101, Speech 101, History 101, Journalism 101. I really haven't gotten many grades yet.

RA: You mean you haven't had any assignments or tests?

Elroy: No, there were some tests and assignments; I just haven't had a chance to turn in my stuff, or I was not in class when the tests were given.

RA: Why haven't you been going to class?

Elroy: I've had other things to do. I have been working extra hard around the fraternity and see joining XX as a once-in-a-lifetime opportunity. I wanted to make sure that I got everything just right. I did talk to some of my teachers. My English teacher doesn't like me. She keeps giving all kinds of stupid assignments that aren't worth my time to do. Last night I was up so late doing things for my fraternity that I decided it would be better for me to sleep-in and get a good night's rest. That is why I missed the quiz in history. I forgot about it. I had some other things to do and didn't go to class the last few times—the professor is real boring. I went to him and asked him if I could do a make-up because I didn't know about the quiz, and he said no. He really doesn't care if I get the information or not. He is being unfair about it.

RA: Is there any chance that you can still salvage this semester based on the assignments you have left to do?

Elroy: Sure, I still have at least 60% of my grade in each of the classes resting on how I do in the next three weeks. I really plan to get down to studying soon. I do my best work when I am under pressure, and I didn't see any reason why I should devote the whole quarter worrying about assignments that aren't due until the end of the quarter. You know college is more than just going to classes.

The RA asks Elroy to make a list of the final exams and papers he has due prior to the end of the quarter. What he has left to complete this semester is the following: Math—two problem solution tests, Speech—one speech and one multiple choice test, English—one essay exam, History—one 20-page term paper on George Washington, and Journalism—two stories of approximately three pages each. After analyzing the assignments, Elroy starts to feel a little panicked. He has so much to do and does not know how or where to begin. Elroy asks his RA to help him organize the last three weeks of the quarter.

Questions

1. Identify the rationalizations Elroy has used to avoid studying.

2. Identify the steps that Elroy needs to undertake to begin the process of studying.

3. To complete the 20 page history paper required of Elroy, the RA suggests that Elroy divide the research and writing of the paper into segments, and do some work on the paper each day. Divide the paper into logical segments and estimate the number days within the three week period (21 days) which you would devote to each segment.

4. What suggestions would you make for how Elroy should complete the two assignments he has yet to complete in Speech (one speech and one multiple choice test)?

5. What suggestions would you make for how Elroy should study for his English assignment (one essay test)?

6. What suggestions would you make for how Elroy should study for his math tests (two problem-solving math tests, total recall)?

A Two Week Vacation

Leona is a very busy RA. She is busy helping everyone with their problems, developing programs for her residents, helping at the main desk, and spending time with the other RAs in the building. She is a very nice person. All the women on her floor like her, and she is one of the most energetic and fun people on the RA staff. She thinks she might want to go to graduate school in student personnel administration after she finishes her bachelors degree.

She has one problem; she is not a good student. Each semester the hall director reminds her that she must have at lease a 2.0 GPA (4.0 = A) each semester to remain an RA. So far, she has made it, but just barely. In truth, she can do the academic work. It is just that she likes being an RA so much more than being a student that she spends all of her time helping others and doing ''RA stuff'' that she puts her studying off and then tries to cram at the last minute.

Two weeks before final exams, Leona begins to study. First she tries to study in her room, but because she is so popular, there is a steady stream of visitors. Not wanting to be rude, she sits and chats with her friends as they come into her room. After three days of this, she decides to go to the library to study. She sets aside each evening from 7:00 P.M. to midnight to study. She finds a place she likes in the library and starts to study but is soon interrupted by people at the next table talking. She wanders the library trying to find the best place to study, but can't seem to get comfortable anywhere.

Eventually, she goes to a friend's apartment off-campus and more or less moves in for the last two weeks of the semester. She figures that she has given the students on her floor all her time up to this point, and from now through finals week they will just have to fend for themselves. She believes that she has more than met her RA obligations in the amount of time she has devoted to the job, and the university owes her the time off at the end of the semester to complete her academic work.

Questions

1. Is Leona justified in leaving her residents to fend for themselves in the last two weeks of the semester? Why or why not?

2. If you were Leona's hall director, what advice would you give her for studying in her room and still being available for the residents on her floor?

3. If you were Leona's hall director, how would you evaluate her overall performance as an RA? Explain your answer.

4. What adjectives would you use to explain Leona's reasoning for delaying studying until the end of the semester and then spending all of her time off-campus studying?

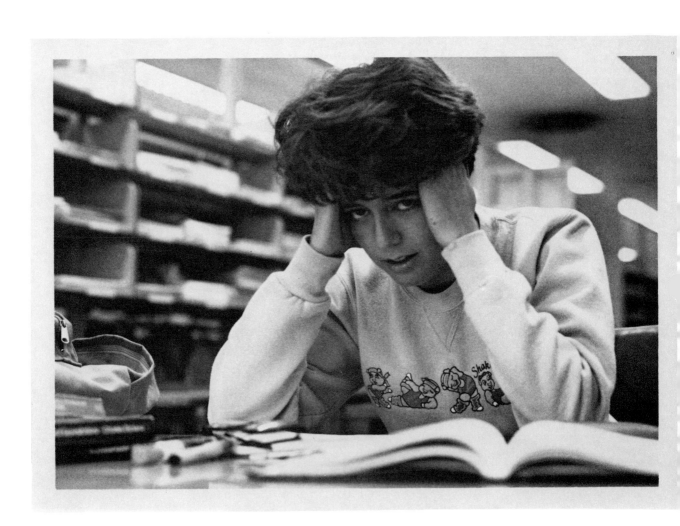

CHAPTER 21

Stress Management

1. What situations do you personally find particularly stressfull?

2. Give two examples of stress that is good for a person.

    1.

    2.

3. What intensifies the reaction to stress?

4. List three of the problems associated with stress.

    1.

    2.

3.

5. Give three ways to reduce or prevent the accumulation of stress.

    1.

    2.

    3.

6. What is the relationship between stress and sleeping patterns?

7. What is the relationship between preventing stress and interpersonal communication?

8. What is "burn-out", and what contributes to it?

9. What steps do you use, or will you use to avoid ''burn-out''?

10. For you, what is, or will be, the most stressful part about being an RA?

Responsibilities

Tracy is a third year RA and will graduate at the end of the semester. Her mind is on graduating and finding a job. She has been interviewing during all of last semester and has not secured a position. Jobs in her field are hard to find. It is particularly difficult for her because she wants to stay in the same city where her boyfriend, Carl, plans to attend law school. Carl will also graduate this semester. Their plan is to get married and for Tracy to find a job and support both of them while Carl goes to law school. When Carl finishes law school and gets a job, Tracy wants to go back to school to get an advanced degree in her field.

Tracy's residents are mostly freshmen, and Tracy is a bit tired of their immaturity. She has lost most of her enthusiasm for the job and had it not been that she needed the money and that it looked good on her resume, she probably wouldn't have stayed on as an RA for a third year. Her residents had all the normal day-to-day problems. One woman had attempted to commit suicide on her floor during mid-terms and was returned to live on the floor after one of the university's psychologists suggested that this was the best decision for the student. Two of the women on the floor were in the middle of breaking-up with their boyfriends, and there was some racial tension mounting among a group of women at one end of the floor. Tracy's hall director was in a automobile accident and would be unable to return to the residence hall for the remainder of the semester. The senior RA, who Tracy did not like very much, was put in charge of the hall, and Tracy had to report to her.

As graduation got closer, Tracy became more self-involved. She got angry over unimportant things and would frequently refuse to answer her door. She looked very tired and had a cold. On several occasions she started to cry for no apparent reason. She had a fight with her boyfriend and had taken to eating compulsively.

Questions

1. Identify the stresses Tracy is under.

2. What are the behavioral signs that she is not coping effectively with the stress?

3. If you were Tracy's best friend, what suggestions would you give her for relieving, or at least coping with, the stress?

4. Some people have argued that RAs should not be hired for a third year. What do you think about having third year RAs?

All That It Can Be

Dak was a new freshmen and wanted college to be everything it could possibly be. His father told him the importance of getting good leadership experience in college, and he wanted his resume at the end of his college career to be as strong as possible. He believed that to succeed in the world he had to be aggressive and put himself and his interests first.

He joined a fraternity, ran for an office in student government, had a work-study job on campus, was the information officer for the College Republicans, and had a girlfriend. There were several other clubs he planned to join, but had not yet done so. His goal was to become the President of the Student Government Association, and to be an officer in enough student organizations to get invited to join the two most prestigious honor societies on campus. He was carrying 18 semester hours, and was doing moderately well (B average) in all of his classes. He was also involved in the residence hall. He was on the residence hall judicial board and was the social chairman for the Residence Hall Association.

Dak was hoping to get an RA job in the second semester of his freshman year to fill one of the vacancies that usually occurs mid-year. He knew it would look good on his resume, and over time, it might give him a better chance at being a senior RA with supervisory experience over some of the other RAs. Dak spent some of his time each day with Leroy, his RA. He also stopped to see the hall director at least twice a week to chat.

The strain of all of these activities was wearing on Dak. He was frequently ill, never seemed to have enough time to sleep, and would come back to his room every night and drink two or three beers. Although this was illegal, only his roommate knew.

Leroy suggested to Dak that he cut back on some of his activities and try to pace himself. Dak told him his father's motto, ''Winners never quit, and quitters never win.'' He couldn't stand to drop any of his activities because he couldn't stand to let his father down.

Questions

1. What three questions would you ask Dak in his RA interview?

    1.

    2.

    3.

2. If Dak were hired as an RA, what would you see as his strengths and weaknesses?

3. Write an end to the above case study based on what you consider to be the most likely outcome for Dak.

4. If you were Leroy, what suggestions would you offer Dak for pacing himself?

5. If Dak were given an RA position, how would you feel about being one of his residents?

Supplemental Case Studies

CASE STUDY 22.1

The Case of the Gay Roommates

As Tom Wagoner and Scott Clark left their room, they were not sure what to expect when they returned. For the past two months, they had endured catcalls, death threats, abusive language, and a daily barrage of laughter, ridicule, and harassment from the other residents on their floor. Tom and Scott were openly gay students. Tom was the president of the gay student alliance, and Scott was a frequent contributor of editorials about gay issues to the student newspaper.

Tom and Scott were both sophomores who came to State University in their freshman year. Tom was an English major, and Scott was majoring in engineering. Both students were good athletes, and both were involved in the university's community service efforts. Tom and Scott met during their freshman year at a meeting of the gay student alliance. They became friends and chose to room together in their sophomore year. Both young men dated other gay students. They chose to room together, not because they were romantically involved with each other, but because they felt more comfortable living with another gay person who understood their lifestyle and with whom each could be open.

Tom's parents accepted his sexual orientation. He had a brother who also was openly gay, and the parents were not surprised when Tom announced to them during his freshman year that he was gay. Scott told his parents that he was gay just before returning to college in his sophomore year. His parents were shocked and angry. They told him that this was a passing phase and he would grow out of it. His mother had written him recently about the daughter of a friend of hers who was attending State University. She was convinced that if he would start dating women, his "confusion" over his sexual orientation would be resolved.

Tom and Scott were sensitive to how the other residents on the floor would react to them when they found out they were gay; but, they believed that it would be too stressful to hide it from others and that they had nothing to be ashamed of.

Bubba Jones was a resident on the same floor with Tom and Scott. One afternoon when he was reading the student newspaper, he read an article written by Scott Clark about gay rights. In the article, it encouraged students who had questions about their sexual orientation to come to one of the first meetings of the gay student alliance. It gave Tom Wagoner's name as the president of the organization and listed their residence hall room as a telephone number to contact for more information. Bubba walked across the hall and showed the article to four other male residents of the hall who were playing cards in the floor lounge. The conversation went like this:

Bubba: "Hey, guys, read this. The two guys at the end of the hall, Tom and Scott, are both fags. I hate fags."

Norman: "You've got to be kidding. I'm not going to be living with any queers. God, I was taking a shower the other day and he was in the bathroom. I'll never let that happen again."

Frank: "I'll bet those two are having sex in their room every night. They probably have AIDS and we're all going to catch it."

Paul: "I'll bet the university doesn't know that this is going on. Surely they'll put a stop to it once they learn that these two students are gay and are messing around with each other in the residence halls. This whole thing grosses me out."

The five men go to the RA, Joe Henry, and inform him of this new information. Joe Henry did not know that Tom and Scott were gay, but he wasn't surprised. He explained that four years ago the university adopted a policy prohibiting discrimination on the basis of sexual orientation, and that during RA training they had a session on gay and lesbian issues. He explained to the residents that these students had a right to be in the residence halls and the university did not consider sexual orientation in the assignment of roommates, just like they did not consider race when assigning roommates. Joe Henry told the students, "I don't like queers any more than anyone else, but the university's philosophy is live and let live."

That night someone scrawled on the outside of Tom and Scott's door the following note: "We don't want any queers on our floor. MOVE OR DIE!" Tom and Scott took the note to the RA and asked him to do something. The RA took it to the hall director, who called the director of residence life. It was decided that the RA should talk with the residents of the floor and determine if anybody knew anything about who did it. No one would say. The next few weeks involved more of the same kinds of behavior. If Tom or Scott would go to the restroom on the floor, the other students would immediately leave. If they walked down the hall, they could hear students laughing at them behind their backs and calling them names. Some would yell sexually explicit remarks.

Joe Henry's efforts to discover who was responsible for the constant harassment of water, shaving cream, fireworks, and urine left under their door on almost a nightly basis was unsuccessful. Glue had been put in their lock, and the outside of their door was scarred and marked with various comments, notes, and threats. It reached the point that Tom and Scott feared for their lives. They couldn't study, the room was a constant target of abuse, and they could no longer tolerate the harassment. Together the students went to see the Dean of Students and explained to him in detail what had transpired. Accompanying them to this meeting was the university's affirmative action officer, part of whose responsibility included insuring that the university's non-discrimination policies—including the prohibition against discrimination on the basis of sexual orientation—was enforced. The Dean of Students listened carefully and assured the young men that he would do everything in his power to see that this behavior stopped. The Dean called a meeting with the Director of Residence Life, the hall director, and Joe Henry, the RA on the floor. Joe Henry informed the group that he had tried hard to locate people responsible for the harassment and the threats but was unsuccessful. Even an investigation by police officers and the hall director was negative in linking specific individuals to specific events. Joe Henry's best guess was that everybody on the floor was involved to some degree.

Questions

1. Select four people and assign to them the following four roles: Dean of students, hall director, resident assistant, and affirmative action officer. Role play the meeting to resolve the problems on Tom and Scott's floor.

2. Design a strategy to stop the harassment of Tom and Scott, keeping in mind that the university has a policy which prohibits discrimination on the basis of sexual orientation and that Tom and Scott are aware of legal rights that they may have if the university fails to take appropriate action.

3. Tom Wagoner's parents call the president of the university and tell her about what transpired. They ask her why she is unable to provide a satisfactory educational environment for their son and suggest that if she can't insure the safety of their son and his right to an education, they will hire an attorney for their son, sue the university, and bring as much public attention through the media and through gay and lesbian organizations as possible to punish the university for its failure to act. If you were the president of the university, how would you respond to Mr. and Mrs. Wagoner and what action, if any, would you take?

Friends and Enemies

Elizabeth and Verdola were African-American students attending Mid-State University. This was their first year in college, and they were nervous about going to a university so far away from home and one that was 95% White students. Their RA was a junior named April. This was her first year as an RA, and she was eager to make friends and get to know all of the students. The residence hall was a suite-style arrangements where two rooms shared a bathroom between them. It so happened that April's room adjoined Elizabeth and Verdola's room. They soon made friends. They usually kept the doors open to the bathroom so that they could easily walk into each other's rooms through the bathroom. Often the women would borrow items from one another's rooms (clothing, jewelry, cosmetics). One afternoon April needed an iron to iron a dress for a date and went next door to borrow Verdola's iron. Neither Elizabeth or Verdola was in, and April took the iron and used it. When she was finished, she unplugged the iron and put it on the window sill behind the curtain and forgot about it.

Elizabeth and Verdola liked rap music and frequently played it at a high volume late into the evening. April on three occasions during the semester asked them to turn down the music, and Verdola and Elizabeth did. One night while April was the duty RA, she was called to the floor by several of her residents because the music coming from Verdola and Elizabeth's room was so loud that no one could sleep. The residents told April that they had spoken with Verdola and Elizabeth but that they refused to turn down their stereo. April knocked on the door, and Elizabeth and Verdola answered it. The conversation went like this:

April: Your stereo is too loud again. I've received several complaints from students on the floor about the noise. You must turn the stereo down.''

Verdola: ''Other people play their stereos loud all the time. You never complain when it's White people's music that is being played.''

Elizabeth: ''The women on this hall don't like us because we're Black. This is just an excuse to try to make us look bad.''

April: ''I've spoken with you several times about how loud your stereo is played. You must keep it down.

Verdola: ''You're just like all the other White people on the floor. You really don't care about us.''

April: ''You've left me no choice. I'm going to have to write an incident report on this and send it to the hall director for appropriate disciplinary action under the hall judicial system.''

Elizabeth: ''If you do that, we'll never speak to you again.''

Verdola: ''I knew you couldn't be trusted.''

At this point Elizabeth and Verdola closed the door and turned down their stereo. April wrote an incident report and sent it to the hall director. The hall director was a Mexican-American man who was working on his doctoral degree in college student personnel administration. His name was Jose.

The students were furious at their RA for writing an incident report and secretly swore that they would get even. Approximately three days after the incident Jose arranged for Verdola and Elizabeth to meet with him in his office. He informed them of the incident and read them the report written by their RA. In part the report said the following:

On Wednesday night at 1:00 a.m. I was called to the room of Elizabeth and Verdola. I knocked on the door and I asked them to turn down their stereo. They refused. Some words were exchanged between us, and they closed the door in my face. Eventually they turned down the stereo. I have had numerous conversations with them about loud noise in the hall, and many of the residents of my floor have complained to me about them. Something needs to be done to get them to act like the rest of the students on the floor and follow residence hall rules.

Elizabeth and Verdola got angry as they listened to the incident report. They informed the hall director that their stereo may have been a little loud but that there was a much deeper problem. Their RA, April, they believed was a racist. Elizabeth and Verdola said that they were the only African-American women on the floor and that everybody on the floor was against them. April was White and she was siding with the other White women on the floor against the only two Black women. Furthermore, they claimed that April had come into their room without their permission and used some of their belongings. Specifically, they claimed that she "snuck in when they weren't there and stole several CDs and an iron." They said that they never gave her permission to use any of these things and, therefore, they wished to file a complaint against her.

Jose said he would look into the matter and that he thought it in the best interest of everyone for him to refer this noise violation to the residence hall judicial board. Elizabeth and Verdola were upset with their meeting and believed that Jose did not understand the situation and that he would side with his RA. They went to the Director of Multicultural Affairs on campus who was an African-American woman employed in the Division of Student Affairs at the university. They told the Director of Multicultural Affairs that the RA, the hall director, and the women on their floor were racists and were mounting a racial attack against them. They said that the reason the women on the floor objected to the music was that they didn't like the kind of music they played and they didn't like them because they were African-American. They also told the Director that their RA had entered their room and taken items without their permission. The Director of Multicultural Affairs was sympathetic and assured the students that she would look into the matter.

As the young women encountered their friends on campus, they began to tell the same story. As the story progressed, it became embellished with other minor incidents that the women said were further evidence of the racism on the floor. Verdola was a member of the campus Black Student Association, and at their meeting that week she brought up the incident as an example of how African-Americans were mistreated on campus. Elizabeth wrote an article in the student newspaper in the "letters to the editor" column describing how the Office of Residence Life was racist because they failed to protect her individual rights and how the staff in the building in which she lived was against her because she was African-American.

By the time the residence hall judicial board was convened to hear their case, many of the African-American students on campus had taken sides supporting Verdola and Elizabeth. They truly believed that Verdola and Elizabeth were the victims of open racism on campus. This incident became symbolic for other incidents that had occurred with African-American students on the campus and was being used as a test to see whether or not African-American students would be treated fairly through the residence hall judicial system.

April, the RA, was feeling somewhat embattled. The other RAs in her building, some of her close friends, and the residence life staff supported her. On campus, the RAs were viewing this situation, which had become increasingly public, as a test to see whether or not the university would support them when they had a conflict with a student.

Questions

1. What do you think the RA could have done differently?

2. What are some of the advantages and disadvantage of RAs developing close personal relationships with the residents on their floor?

3. Do you believe it is reasonable for Verdola and Elizabeth to perceive this as a racial issue?

4. Given the emotion and publicity around this incident, do you believe the university officials should intercede to resolve the situation before a decision is made by the residence hall judicial board?

5. If you were on the residence hall judicial board and had to make a decision about what to do in this situation, how would you decide based on the information in the case?

The Hopeful Freshman

Lester was a brand new freshman at a small private liberal arts college of approximately 2000 students located in the Midwest. He was excited about being accepted to this college. Both his mother and father were graduates of the college, and it had an excellent academic reputation. The college was pleased to have Lester as a freshman. He had good SAT scores, good grades, and the college liked having the children of alumni at the institution.

The college held orientation and preregistration during the middle of the summer. Lester was unable to attend over the summer because he was vacationing with his grandparents on a European excursion that they had planned as part of his high school graduation gift. The college offered orientation again at the beginning of the fall semester, and Lester planned to attend that orientation.

The day the residence hall opened, Lester was there with his parents and moved into his room. He was assigned to live on a floor that was composed of students approximately 80% of whom were members of a fraternity called Chi Lambda Alpha. His RA was not a member of the fraternity and was in his first year of being an RA. Because the residence halls opened on Saturday and many of the college offices were not open, Lester was not able to get his student ID or eat in the cafeteria under the meal plan until Monday. He knew this before coming and had brought some additional money with him to purchase food from some of the restaurants near the campus. He attended the orientation sessions; however, between the testing for class, preregistration and the regular fall orientation that all students went through, he missed various sessions and felt like there was too much to learn in too short of a time.

Within approximately two days, all of the residents of his floor had arrived. The RA had the first floor meeting. At that meeting he said:

"I want everyone to get along on this floor this year. It is more important to me that we have a sense of community and do things together than anything else. The college requires that I enforce certain policies as part of my job, but I'm not going to be a 'super sleuth.' I know a lot of you like to drink beer, which is in violation of college policy. If I don't see it, you won't get in trouble. Drugs are a different matter. If you have drugs on the floor, you are going to get caught and the university will suspend you from school. Just be cool with the alcohol and no one is going to hassle you."

That night there was a spontaneous floor party. Most of the students were drinking beer. The RA was nowhere to be found. Lester did not drink. There had been a car accident involving some close friends of his in high school who were killed by a drunk driver, and Lester had become involved with a high school student organization dedicated to informing students about the hazards of alcohol. He told his mother and father that he was not going to drink while he was in college and, frankly, did not like the taste of beer.

While Lester was in his residence hall room unpacking, one of the members of Chi Lambda Alpha came into his room and said, "Why aren't you partying with the guys?" Lester explained that he didn't drink. The student said, "Only sissies don't drink; and, if you want to be a member of this floor, you're going to have to learn to drink or we'll make life miserable for you. We don't want any guys associated with our fraternity who aren't man enough to have a beer with the guys." Lester asked the student to leave his room and leave him alone. Some words were exchanged between the two students, and the fraternity member pushed Lester, who pushed him back. The fraternity member said he better keep his door locked because the next time he saw him he was going to beat him to a bloody pulp.

Lester closed his door and locked it. He was frightened. He knew that the fraternity had some big guys in it and that he couldn't stand to live on the floor wondering if he was going to get beaten up. His dreams about what college life was going to be like were shattered. He felt disoriented, confused, unaccepted by the residents of his own floor, and in an environment where alcohol was everywhere. He called his parents and told them the whole story. He said that he feared for his life. His parents advised him to leave the residence hall and to go to a friend of theirs who lived in the community. By morning, Lester decided that he had made a mistake about the college and wanted nothing more to do with it.

Questions

1. What could the RA have done to assist in this situation?

2. Do you believe that there is a lot of pressure placed on students to drink and that students who do not drink are often ostracized by other students?

3. Given that there are no other rooms available to place students, what do you think the college can do to help Lester?

4. On Monday morning, Lester's parents call the director of residence life and tell her what happened. Do you think that the director of residence life should fire the RA or take some other disciplinary action against him?

5. Is there anything that could have been done to train the RA that would have helped him do a better job with his residents?

6. What do you think of the idea of having fraternities and sororities assigned to live on residence hall floors knowing that any vacancies that occur will have to be filled by non-fraternity or sorority students?